CHILDHOOD INTERRUPTED

CHILDHOOD INTERRUPTED

The Complete Guide to PANDAS and PANS

Pediatric **A**utoimmune **N**europsychiatric **D**isorders **A**ssociated with **S**treptococcal Infections

Pediatric **A**cute-onset **N**europsychiatric **S**yndrome

by Beth Alison Maloney
author of *Saving Sammy:
Curing the Boy Who Caught OCD*

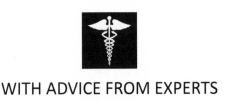

WITH ADVICE FROM EXPERTS

DEDICATION

This book is dedicated to:

my sons
Josh, Sammy, and James.

Rebecca Craighill Lancefield, Ph.D.
(January 5, 1895 – March 3, 1981),
a mother and scientist from the past who devoted her
lifelong career to unraveling the biology of strep.

Tanya K. Murphy, M.D.
of the University of South Florida,
a mother and treating physician whose PANDAS
research is leading us into the future.

CONTENTS

Think too deeply about what you're doing
and the enormity of the thing can stop you from getting it done.

Jeffrey Kluger

Introduction: Solving Our Puzzle

When my middle son, Sammy, was twelve years old he was suddenly struck with an increasingly bizarre series of behaviors, just before the start of sixth grade. He was diagnosed first with obsessive-compulsive disorder, next Tourette's, and then I was told that he might be in and out of hospitals for the rest of his life. He went from totally normal to completely dysfunctional in the space of weeks while doctors shook their heads and prescribed increasing doses of psychotropic medications that never helped. Confined to our home by the severity of his illness, his world shrank to a couch in our den. Month after month passed as I struggled to come to terms with the illness that had come out of nowhere. I kept asking doctors to explain what had happened. He'd been a completely normal boy until he turned twelve.

"It happens," I was told.

Sammy was sick for a full year before I found the missing piece of the puzzle: a link between strep, OCD, and tics. Another mom told me about it. No doctor had ever mentioned the possibility that perhaps Sammy had caught something that was making him mentally ill. We ran a simple blood test, and there it was with startling clarity. The results showed that an elevated level of strep antibodies surged through his system. His brain was under attack. The disorder is called PANDAS: Pediatric Autoimmune Neuropsychiatric Disorders Associated with Streptococcal Infections.

I thought that was the end of our journey, but it was only the beginning. It was extremely difficult to find treatment. Doctors dismissed the link between his infection and his mental illness.

Even with blood work indicating strep, doctors said there was no connection.

"The best thing you can do for your son," said a well-respected pediatric neurologist in Boston, "is to take him home and accept the diagnosis of OCD."

Instead of doing that, I redoubled my efforts. I located a physician with the correct expertise; she was four hundred miles away. Month after month, we made the trek from Maine to southern New Jersey to see Catherine Nicolaides, MD, a developmental pediatrician. Sammy would lie across the back seat of my van, too weak to move. He had already missed all of sixth grade and the start of seventh grade. But after a few visits he could ride sitting up and, a few months later, banter with his brother as we drove. Under Dr. Nicolaides' tender care and guidance, along with the insight of Boston psychiatrist Daniel Geller, MD, to whom Dr. Nicolaides referred us, slowly and steadily Sammy began to recover. With appropriate antibiotic treatment (Augmentin XR), a gradually reduced prescription of psychotropic medications, and cognitive behavioral therapy, Sammy was finally able to rejoin his classmates in eighth grade. It took four full years of antibiotics taken every day for the disorder to be fully treated. And for two years after that he occasionally had compulsions when he was exposed to strep. But by the time Sammy entered college, he was fully recovered and took no medication at all. He has now graduated from Carnegie Mellon University with a degree in computer science and mathematics: no meds, no behaviors, just fully recovered. The future is brilliant for this young man who had been destined to be in and out of mental treatment facilities for the rest of his life.

Saving Sammy: Curing the Boy Who Caught OCD was published by Random House in 2009. I was determined that no one would suffer as we had. *Saving Sammy* is my memoir recounting those painful years as we battled to find an appropriate diagnosis and treatment. More important, it is a story of ultimate triumph. Following publication, I made scores of media appearances for which Sammy often joined me. I spoke at conferences, met with the deans of medical schools, compiled lists of treatment providers, spearheaded the formation of support groups, and generally demanded action as word of PANDAS began to spread. Organizations devoted to the recognition and treatment of PANDAS popped up across the country. Thousands of e-mails began pouring in from parents with similar stories of heartbreak, most of whom previously had no idea that they should wonder about an undiagnosed infection.

What those parents needed was guidance. Thus was born the idea for this book. Their thousands of individual stories had common themes: the hopelessness of not knowing where to turn, the difficulty in finding treatment, the desperation and frustration of not finding answers, and the wondering what to do on a daily basis. Their stories and questions are woven anonymously throughout this book.

As I write, this area of medicine is still finding its way. There is not yet a published protocol for the treatment of PANDAS (much less PANS), which was originally reported in the late 1990s. Doctors remain skeptical. Parents, trapped in a sea of confusion, are dismissed as overreacting. Reports of children responding to antibiotics are dismissed as "anecdotal." But the bright spots glow stronger. The NIMH has stopped referring to PANDAS as "rare." It has also broadened the diagnostic criteria for PANDAS and acknowledged that many physicians believe antibiotic therapy is an effective form of treatment for the disorder. Moreover, PANS is now proposed on its website. The International OCD Foundation (IOCDF) has included PANDAS on its website. It has also released two PSAs alerting doctors to the fact that an infection should be considered whenever a child presents with a behavioral disorder. Michael Jenike, MD, chair of the IOCDF's scientific advisory board, has stated openly that he believes the disorder is not rare, but rather rarely diagnosed.

This book pushes through the confusion. It is a common-sense reference guide that will help streamline the complicated process of grappling with PANDAS by offering a roadmap for recognition, treatment, and recovery. It covers all the information that I needed and could not find when my son was desperately ill, so grab a highlighter and dig in.

I'm not a doctor, and I'm not a researcher. I'm a lawyer and a mom sharing what I've learned, and you should not consider anything in this book as medical advice. What I hope is that you will consider whether an infection may be the root cause of any mental health issue that a child is experiencing. Infection will not be the answer in every case, but the greatest news I ever received was to learn that Sammy had strep. It changed the course of our lives. Hopefully, the information in this book will change yours, too.

Whatever you do, don't give up when you get discouraged: reach out for help, rest when you need to, but just keep going. You are the CEO of your child's life, and it's the most important position you will ever hold.

Beth Alison Maloney

CHILDHOOD INTERRUPTED

I

UNDERSTANDING PANDAS AND PANS

What Is PANDAS/PANS?

PANDAS stands for Pediatric Autoimmune
Neuropsychiatric Disorders Associated with
Streptococcal Infections.

In a nutshell, researchers believe that PANDAS occurs when strep antibodies attack the brain and produce behaviors. The presence of a strep infection correlates with the presence of the behavioral disorder.

PANDAS is not as new and controversial as you might be told. Descriptions of infections triggering disturbing behaviors began as early as the 1800s. In the 1920s, reports linked the behaviors to sinusitis. In the 1950s, strep was linked to the movement disorder Sydenham's Chorea. And in the late 1990s, PANDAS was officially identified. In 2011, the NIMH proposed criteria for a much broader, related disorder known as PANS: Pediatric Acute-onset Neuropsychiatric Syndrome. PANS proposes that behavioral disorders can be triggered by a number of infections, not just strep. This book will most often refer to PANDAS because it is a more established diagnosis, but the principles of the two disorders are basically the same. If you understand PANDAS, you will also be able to understand PANS.

Why It's Confusing

One of the confusing things is that PANDAS and PANS don't fit into our framework of what to expect from an infection. We think of strep as giving our children sore throats and temperatures. We may remember hearing that a relative had rheumatic fever and heart problems that were caused by strep. We might even have heard news reports about an unusual case of strep that attacked the skin. Those all fit within the common understanding of what an infection does: it makes us physically ill in the traditional sense. What isn't widely known or accepted is that sometimes a child's concerning behaviors can be symptoms of strep or another infection. And that's part of what this chapter is about: *recognizing the different behaviors that may be symptoms of an infection and trusting ourselves* when we know we need to search further for what is causing those behaviors.

We need to trust our instincts when it comes to PANDAS because nothing about it is black and white. Medicine is just at the beginning of recognizing this disorder, so PANDAS is still in its infancy. There isn't a checklist yet for whether your child has PANDAS, and there isn't an established protocol or a series of easy diagnostic steps to follow. If your child's behaviors are concerning, and you are not satisfied with the answers you have received to explain those behaviors, then you are right to wonder if an infection might be the root cause of what's troubling your child. What you are doing is following your instincts. They guide us every day. They help us choose friends, avoid strangers, and know when a problem is looming. Instincts are what enable us to sometimes know what our children want or need before they do. Our instincts gnaw at us when we know something is wrong, but we can't put our finger on it. Instincts help us sort through confusing situations.

FACT:

Part of being a good parent is trusting our instincts.

This helps explain another odd thing about PANDAS: parents are often the first to raise PANDAS as a possibility. We usually look to doctors to guide us regarding health concerns. If you think it through, though, it's not necessarily surprising that parents may be the first to mention PANDAS. We take our children to the doctor when we suspect a strep or ear infection. We take them when their bellies won't stop aching. We take them when we spot a rash or a tick bite. Parents are the first to wonder about their child's well-being because they know their child better than anyone else. So when parents don't feel that they have found the answer to what's troubling their child, they may suggest PANDAS. Generally it's because the children are acting so differently from the past. Friends and relatives may reassure us that the child is simply going through a rough patch or will "grow out of it," but our instincts cause us to wonder. If you wonder whether there might be another explanation for what is going on with your child, or if you absolutely know that all is not well, then you are two steps ahead because you are already questioning. Asking questions is part of being a PANDAS parent. Being brave enough to ask the questions may take some practice, but by reading this book you have already taken the first step to acquiring the knowledge you need.

Keep in mind that your pediatrician sees hundreds of children. Your attention is focused only on yours. While many doctors are willing to help, they may not know what to do and are often under a great deal of pressure. It's possible that by the end of this book you will know more about PANDAS than your child's own doctor, so don't be shy about sharing what you learn. Knowing the behaviors that may indicate a future problem will help sharpen your instincts.

How Children Might Behave When They Have It

There are behavioral symptoms that suggest your child may have an underlying infection. If you don't recognize them, then your child's infection may go undiagnosed and untreated. For that reason, you need to know which behaviors can be the early signs of an infection. And if your child is one whose behaviors are the clue that he may have an infection, you will need to keep a careful eye so that you can immediately intervene if the infection returns after proper treatment.

The Early Signs Suggesting PANDAS/PANS

There are some children who will suddenly have a full-blown tornado of behaviors. They happily drift off to sleep one night and wake up the next day a totally different, unmanageable child. But their parents and the doctors who treat them say that, in retrospect, there were early behavioral hints, or *soft signs*, along the way that a bigger problem was brewing. These soft signs, sometimes called *micro-episodes*, are behaviors that are new or unexpected for a child, but still manageable. They whisper that a problem may be coming.

What the doctor says:

"There may be some minor behaviors in the background, perhaps even for years, which suddenly explode. It's as if someone abruptly turns up the volume to an excruciating level."

David Band, MD
Crossroads Psychological Associates
Columbia, MD and Ashburn, VA

Any of the behavioral changes listed below may be soft signs of PANDAS. If your child is experiencing any of these difficulties, and especially a combination of more than one, you want to make it a point to notice whether they are becoming more prominent.

Obsessions

Compulsions

Tics

Regressions

Touch, hearing, sight, taste, and
  smell issues

Refusal to eat

Inability to concentrate

Impulsivity/distraction

Separation anxiety

Bedtime fears

Rapid mood swings

Episodes of stuttering

Raging, sobbing, screaming

Threatening or worrying about
  harm

Irritability

Sleep disturbance

Urination issues

Changes in handwriting

Joint pain—consider also
  rheumatic fever,
  rheumatoid disorder, or
  Lyme disease

Personality changes at home
  and/or school

Abnormal movements, sometimes called "choreiform movements," may indicate PANDAS, but their presence should always cause consideration of whether the child may have rheumatic fever or another neurological disorder. Such movements may include jerking, writhing, lack of coordination, tics, and twitching (myoclonus).

Three Examples of Early Signs

Parents report that many PANDAS children have separation anxiety, get stuck and regress, or have tics. Some children may have all three together. Because these three are some of the most common behaviors, I am using them as examples. All the behaviors listed above may grow into much bigger problems, but these offer a good illustration. And I chose separation anxiety to more fully describe how an early sign might escalate from difficult into something far more challenging and disabling.

Separation Anxiety: Ordinarily, when our children don't feel well, they don't like us to leave them. They want mom around to put a cold cloth on their foreheads and kiss their sick tummies. They want dad to tell them a special story. They'd rather not be left with a babysitter. They want you. This is all normal behavior. Suppose though that your second-grade daughter had what seemed like a minor cold two weeks ago. She's clingier this year than she was last year, but still loves going to school and went even while a bit under the weather with her cold. This week she suddenly does not want to go at all. She says her clothes are uncomfortable; they don't "feel right." None of your suggestions make her happy. It takes her two hours, but she finally gets dressed and agrees to go to school. When it's time for you to leave her there, the teacher has to peel her off you as she sobs. She can't be consoled. You're upset and confused. The teacher wonders if something is going on at home.

Your fears fade when your daughter is back to her old self in a matter of days. She's enjoying school and playing with her friends. But what if it happens again three months later in a much bigger way? This time she refuses to go to school. She screams and cries, and there is no amount of persuasion that will change her mind. You stay home with her because she is so upset. She won't leave your side, not even when you need to use the bathroom. She cries all day. Now you start to question what is really going on. Could it be related to what happened three months ago? Was it just a cold that she had? Could she have PANDAS? Maybe, because a PANDAS child will often have a series of behavioral episodes over the course of childhood. Usually each episode is more extreme than the last and that is called an *exacerbation*.

It's more difficult to track behavioral patterns in younger children.

In very young children it's especially important to be alert to behavioral patterns because those children lack a long-established history. Not many people know a young child well, so it's easy to attribute changes to personal growth. If you have a kindergartener who suddenly starts demonstrating extreme separation anxiety and wets the bed at night, the logical explanation is that your kindergartner is anxious about school. The other possible explanation may be that these are often overlooked signs of an infection. Left unchecked, an infection can become quite serious.

Getting Stuck/Regression: Another sign to look for is whether your child is getting "stuck." Each child is different, but it seems the simplest tasks, the ones taken for granted, have become difficult. The child regresses. You find yourself looking at your child and thinking, "This just isn't like him."

Each child has his or her own version of getting stuck or regressing, but here are some "before" and "now" examples.

A child who...
raced out the door, now can't leave.
regularly washed up before dinner, now can't touch the faucet.
was a good eater, now doesn't like what you
    serve.
wrote clearly, now has trouble writing.
loved school, now doesn't want to go.
spoke clearly, now stutters.
was toilet trained, now wets the bed.
zipped through homework, now can't finish due to painfully
    rechecking.

While getting stuck may be manageable in the beginning, it can grow to become disabling. Checking and rechecking may progress to the point that it's hard for your child to leave the house because there are so many things that she must do first. You never want it to get to that point. This is why knowing the early signs helps.

Tics: Another way that strep can present itself may be a motor or verbal tic. Tics can present themselves in a number of different ways and are four times as likely to show up in boys. Some of the most common are:

Eye blinking	Snorting	Neck rolling
Facial grimaces	Tapping	Head jerking
Coughing		

Even sneezing can be a tic, but the other tics are far more prevalent.

The presence of a tic may indicate a neurological problem, but tics can also be the sign of a strep infection. Often when parents raise concerns about tics to the pediatrician, the doctor feels the child will grow out of it. Sometimes that does happen, but even if a persistent tic is mild and does not significantly impact daily life, it should be taken seriously. For example, sneezing is something that we do occasionally but not repeatedly for hours. A persistent sneeze indicates a problem. You want to make sure there's no infection because you don't want it to escalate to the point that your child is sneezing every few seconds.

Beyond the Early Signs

When an early sign becomes concerning, it may indicate that this is more than a phase the child is going through. Listed below are ten broad categories of behaviors that have been linked to PANDAS. If your child has an increasing level of behaviors within these categories, you want to make sure there is no underlying infection that has gone undetected. Pay special attention if you have a son because PANDAS is particularly prevalent in boys. Pre-puberty OCD affects about three times as many boys as girls, although practitioners report that it is recently on the rise among girls.

After each category of behavior, there is an overview of how the symptoms might present

FACT: PANDAS and OCD are generally thought to affect more boys than girls.

themselves in a PANDAS child. The overviews are not intended to be all-encompassing. There are entire books, websites, and forums devoted to each of these categories that you may want to consult. The two categories of behaviors that account for a large number of PANDAS children are obsessive-compulsive disorder (OCD) and those with motor and verbal tics. For that reason OCD and tics are presented first in this list. The rest of the categories are presented in alphabetical order.

1. *Obsessive-Compulsive Disorder:* OCD can include repetitive behaviors, excessive fear of germs, unwanted thoughts, hoarding, hair pulling, and eating disorders. There are often a set of "rules" that dictate the behaviors, and those rules may prohibit the child from discussing the behaviors.

What might this look like? The child gets stuck and may continue to repeat the same phrase over and over, or become obsessed with particular numbers, colors, items, sounds, or symmetry (keeping things even). His eating pattern suddenly changes. He may fear contamination of his food, his clothes, even the air. Your child may only want to breathe in certain places, so he may hold his breath a lot. He may have cramped hands (piano fingers) or blow on his fingertips. He may fear contracting a fatal disease; blood-related diseases such as AIDS seem to be at the top of the list. Your formerly healthy eater may have eating issues, needing to chew each piece of food a certain number of times, or in a certain way, or he may not be able to eat at all. Overwhelming significance may be inexplicably given to nondescript objects or events. Door handles, faucets, utensils, and chairs may suddenly become untouchable items. Your child may become preoccupied with hygiene, washing his hands until they are raw. He may refuse to leave the house because he might get sick from the germs outside. He may have to walk in patterns or do things until they "feel right." He may have to jump lines endlessly to make certain he didn't miss any of them. He may not be able to go for car rides. He may stand in one place and spin. He may want you to participate in what seem to be senseless rituals. He may start hair pulling: eyelashes, eyebrows, or hair (trichotillomania). He may scratch and pick at his skin.

2. *Motor and Verbal Tics (Tourette's):* When a child has only a motor tic, it is called a tic disorder. A Tourette's diagnosis requires the presence of both motor and verbal (phonic) tics for at least one year.

What might this look like? *Motor tics* may be simple or complex. *Simple tics* show up as twitches and spasms that may include trembling, eye blinking, sneezing, and sniffing. *Complex tics* are "bigger." They include bending, grimacing, shrugging, jaw chomping, and neck rolling. They can interfere with walking. *Vocal tics* usually show up as coughing, grunting, yelping, barking, or throat clearing. Shouting swear words (*copralalia*) receives much attention, but rarely occurs. Those who are afflicted with tics sometimes describe them as an itch that needs to be scratched. Many of the children diagnosed with Tourette's also have OCD behaviors (about one-third) and ADHD (about one-half). Sometimes tics are attributed to being a side effect of ADHD medication, but that may not always be correct.

> *FACT:*
> *Boys are four times more likely than girls to have tics.*

3. Attention Deficit Hyperactivity Disorder (ADHD): ADHD includes hyperactivity, inattention, impulsivity, and fidgety behaviors that are out of the normal range for the child's age and development.

What might this look like? The child may be constantly distracted. She may not be able to sit still, concentrate, or finish school assignments. She may run or climb when she shouldn't and may not be able to play quietly. She may appear to daydream or "zone out." She may get frustrated or bored easily. She may be disorganized and lose things, or make careless errors. These behaviors must be measured against the appropriate expectations for the child's age. While a four-year-old might not be able to sit for prolonged periods of time, a twelve-year-old should be able to do so. If you think your child's level of immaturity or silliness is extreme when compared to others her age, listen to your instinct.

4. Enuresis (Involuntary Urination): Nighttime bedwetting (*nocturnal enuresis*) or constantly having to urinate during the daytime (*pollakiuria*).

What might this look like? A formerly toilet-trained child might suddenly start

> *A new onset of bedwetting should be one of the biggest red flags to a pediatrician that the child may be experiencing a first episode of PANDAS.*

wetting the bed or one who wets the bed may have an increasing problem. It is estimated that 15 percent of eleven-year-old boys have problems with bedwetting (particularly if there is that history with the father), so remember you are looking for a change in patterns. The fact that a child is having difficulty with bedwetting does not necessarily indicate a possible infection. But a formerly trained child who now wets his bed, or is constantly using the toilet during the day, may be at risk.

5. Fine/Gross Motor Changes (Dysgraphia): One consistent barometer seems to be a change in handwriting.
What might this look like? A child who could write legibly can only deliver scribbles. A child who could draw an accurate rendition of a microscope, precisely identifying each particular part, can only mark a few lines down on the page before giving up.

6. Joint Pains: The child's knees, ankles, and elbows may ache.
What might this look like? A child who formerly liked to run and play no longer wants to participate due to leg or other joint pain. While this may be a sign of PANDAS when occurring in the context of behavioral changes, keep in mind that these types of pains may indicate another problem, such as rheumatic fever or Lyme disease.

7. Mood Changes: This includes irritability, sadness, and emotional lability.
What might this look like? The child may cry, scream, and fly into a rage. His behaviors are explosive and out of control. He may try to jump out of a moving car, run away from home, throw things, shout, and yell. She may say she is going to hurt herself, you, other caregivers, siblings, teachers, and peers. Her moods may shift rapidly. She may be screaming about how sad she is feeling.

8. Sensory Defensiveness: A child reacts negatively to sensory input that is ordinarily considered harmless.
What might this look like? This can affect any one or all five of the senses. Your child cannot make eye contact. Lights bother her. She can't stand to hear herself chew. She screams if you touch her. She says her clothes are uncomfortable. She can't tolerate the way food tastes. She says things "smell bad."

9. Separation Anxiety: Extreme clinging and weepiness when it's time to separate from caregivers.

What might this look like? The child does not want to leave your side. She wants to follow you into the bathroom. She stands outside the door and sobs if you insist on your privacy. She stops sleeping in her own bed and wants to sleep only in yours, with you, all the time. She does not want you to leave her at school or with a babysitter and tries to block the door when you attempt to leave. When the teacher or babysitter finally peels her off and you leave, she doesn't regroup to have a fine day once you're gone. She continues to fall apart.

10. Sleep Disturbances: The child sleeps fitfully, if at all.

What might this look like? The child may awaken constantly during the night, toss and turn, pace the house, or lie in bed unable to fall asleep. While sleeping, the child may have jerky motor tics. Verbal tics may cause him to yelp in his sleep.

Comorbid Conditions

Whenever a child has two or more disorders at the same time, doctors call the conditions *comorbid*. It is the medical term for concurrent or co-occurring. One disorder does not have to be the cause of the second disorder for them to be comorbid. It only means they occur together. As mentioned earlier, many patients with Tourette's also have OCD. When they co-occur, the two disorders are called comorbid. As you consider comorbid disorders, it's important to reflect on how they may interrelate if PANDAS is in the mix. OCD and anorexia are often comorbid. But treating a child for an eating disorder, while not understanding that her OCD may be causing her not to eat, will get you nowhere. We've all heard that concern over physical appearance is the primary issue with anorexia. Perhaps, instead, the patient's afraid of germs, or can't stand the sound her jaw makes while chewing. And maybe a strep infection is driving her OCD.

> *FACT: Comorbid conditions are two behavioral disorders that occur together.*

The other comorbid conditions to consider for a PANDAS child are:

OCD and Depression: Depression will be the logical consequence of a child suffering with OCD so debilitating that the poor little guy can't even leave the house. Would you feel bouncy and bright if this happened to you?

OCD and ADHD: Any child will be distracted and unable to concentrate if she has to remain focused only on completing a series of compulsions.

Tourette's and ADHD: Concentration will certainly be challenging if a child has to constantly grunt, throat clear, blink his eyes, and shrug his shoulders.

Overlooked Signs

There are eight other diagnoses and conditions that should cause parents to question whether their child may be plagued by an infection. These diagnoses are sometimes given when PANDAS is present but overlooked. If your child is diagnosed with one or more of these, you might want to consider whether an underlying infection may be present. Again there is a wealth of separate information available about each of these disorders, but this gives you an overview.

1. Autism: Autism is a developmental disorder that affects social and communication skills. Once a child is diagnosed with autism, parents find that virtually every difficult behavior the child experiences is then attributed to the disorder. Therefore, to the extent certain behaviors may be caused by PANDAS, it's never explored but it should be, especially in regressive presentations.

2. Bipolar Disorder: Bipolar disorder used to be known as manic depression. A person with bipolar disorder experiences mood swings that range from extreme highs (mania) to extreme lows (depression). Many children with extreme irritability are diagnosed as bipolar so now the DSM-5 (see chapter 3) has "mood dysregulation disorder."

3. Depression: Depression is when apathy or sad feelings do not pass within a few days and interfere with the daily life of the child and those who care about him. Minor depression is characterized by symptoms that last more than two weeks and interfere with daily functioning. Major depression is completely disabling. Depression presents itself differently in younger children than teenagers.

4. Dysthymia: Dysthymia is long-term depression (two or more years) that prevents normal functioning and may include episodes of major depression.

5. General Anxiety Disorder: GAD is when worry gets out of control. Patients experience chronic anxiety, exaggerated worry, and tension, even when there is little or nothing to provoke these. Their worries are accompanied by physical symptoms, especially fatigue, headaches, muscle tension, muscle aches, difficulty swallowing, trembling, twitching, irritability, sweating, and hot flashes.

6. Learning Disabilities: Learning disabilities affect a child's ability to learn in the same way and at the same rate as other children because their brains receive and process information differently. Learning disabilities can be present in reading, writing, and mathematics. Dyslexia is an example of a reading disability.

7. Oppositional Defiant Disorder: ODD is childhood misbehavior taken to extraordinary levels. It's an ongoing pattern of defiance and disobedience, full of tantrums and anger.

8. Other Autoimmune Disorders: Autoimmune disorders often run in families. If the child or the child's family has a history of autoimmune disorders, particularly rheumatic fever, the child is potentially more at risk for PANDAS. Other examples of autoimmune disorders are: celiac disease, Hashimoto's, lupus, scleroderma, and—rarely—Guillain-Barre syndrome.

SUMMING IT UP

You want to become familiar with the signs indicating PANDAS because the best scenario is, of course, to catch this early. If not, the behaviors may progress to the point that the child is diagnosed with a behavioral disorder, a neurological condition, or a psychiatric

What the doctor says:

"I've been in psychiatry for 20 twenty years, and I've never seen psychotropic medications turn a child around as quickly as I've seen antibiotics turn a PANDAS child around."

Tanya Murphy, MD
University of South Florida

condition. Perhaps the child might even be placed on *psychotropic medication* (the medications prescribed to treat psychiatric conditions). It is true that behavioral symptoms may increase to the point that they become a psychiatric condition. But if your child has an underlying infection, your goal is to find appropriate treatment *before* things become that serious.

Think of it this way: If you have a deep cut on your finger and it becomes infected, a bandage will cover the sore but it won't heal the wound. The wound needs to be properly cleaned and tended. In a PANDAS child, psychotropic medications are comparable to that bandage. They may mask the symptoms, but not address the underlying problem. No doctor would recommend ignoring a wound, so why neglect an infection? And if your child is already on psychotropic medication, but not responding, an infection may be the reason.

Strep is easy to recognize when your child tells you that she has a sore throat and then a rapid throat swab turns up positive, but it's not always that simple. Sometimes your child's behaviors are what let you know there's an infection. This is why being tuned in to your child's behaviors is so important. Your child might never show the traditional symptoms of strep and, even if you suspect it, a throat swab might give a false negative. Or your child may have had a previous strep infection that needs further attention. Usually a pediatrician will prescribe a ten-day course of antibiotics for strep throat, but sometimes the infection requires additional treatment. Infections can linger when not fully treated, even though you gave your child the full prescription. So when you notice a concerning behavioral change, it's wise to consider whether it might indicate the presence of strep or another infection. And always be sure to give your child the fully prescribed course of antibiotics. Don't stop early because the child "seems to feel better."

BIG IDEAS FROM CHAPTER ONE

❑ PANDAS is a newly recognized disorder so things are not yet clear.
❑ We do know that behaviors and tics may be symptoms of a strep infection.
❑ You are the person who knows your child best.
❑ Trust your instincts if you think something is wrong.
❑ Pay attention to behavioral patterns.
❑ PANDAS and OCD are more prevalent in boys than girls.
❑ Tics are present in four times as many boys as girls.
❑ There are ten broad categories of behaviors that may indicate PANDAS, and eight diagnoses and conditions that should also cause a parent to think about PANDAS.
❑ Comorbid conditions are diseases or disorders that occur at the same time.
❑ When a child is failing to respond to psychotropic medicine, that may indicate PANDAS.
❑ Always give your child the fully prescribed course of an antibiotic.

How Can an Infection
Change Behaviors?

2

The essence of PANDAS is that antibodies for Group A strep (the same bacteria that cause sore throats) cross into the brain and attack the basal ganglia. The basal ganglia is the area of the brain that controls behaviors. To really understand PANDAS, it's helpful to understand the basics of infections and how our bodies respond to fight them. I was never much of a biology student, so it wasn't until my son Sammy became sick that I learned how it all works.

The basic concepts about infections are first explained below, including some medical terms. Doctors speak their own language. The more you can follow their concerns, the more effective you will be at advocating for a sick child. After covering infections in general, I explain how the brain can be affected by infections and then how PANDAS became recognized as a unique disorder.

Understanding the information in this chapter will help you more easily follow your child's progress and talk knowledgeably with the doctors. Some of this is complicated, so take your time and use a highlighter to mark the points you find important. If the information feels overwhelming, just skip it for now and move to a different chapter. You can always come back later.

The Basics of Infection

FACT:
Pathogens are the bacteria and viruses that make us sick.

What Causes Infections? Infections are caused by bacteria, viruses, spirochetes, and fungi. These *microbes* (living things) are so tiny that they can only be seen with a microscope. We always have these floating around in our bodies. They are usually either harmless or helpful. But the ones that cause the infections that make us sick are *pathogenic*. I think of these *pathogens* as invaders, but the medical term for them is *"antigen."* An antigen is any foreign substance that triggers the production of *antibodies*.

How Do We Fight Infections? When you think about what is going on in our bodies during an infection, picture a war—the pathogens against the antibodies. When we get sick, our *immune system* sounds off an alarm and rapidly produces antibodies to fight the infection. Antibodies are the body's war troops, deployed by the immune system to fight the invader. If all goes well and our immune system works properly, our antibodies slaughter the invaders, we get better, and the immune system stops producing antibodies. The antibodies that are in our system, which are proteins, degenerate over time. The body rests while the immune system remains alert and ready to defend against the next invader. But sometimes things do not go according to plan. For example, our immune system might not be strong enough to fight (think of a tired soldier). It might be weakened from fighting another infection, which is why we're more susceptible to picking up another "bug" when we're just getting over the flu. Or the invader may be bacteria that are simply too strong for our body to tackle alone. We may need the help of an antibiotic to fight it off. Generally, though, nothing can help with a virus. Tamiflu is an exception when given in the earliest days of the flu. Most viruses though, such as the common cold, have to run their course. And as with any war, the process of winning can be exhausting.

What Is a Titer? A titer is a measure of antibodies in our blood stream so it fluctuates depending upon whether we've had an infection. There are many different types of antibodies because the ones we produce are specific for each infection. A blood test—it's called a titer test—can measure the level of antibodies that are circulating, and that level will let us know if our body has fought a recent infection. If the result is "an elevated titer" or "high titer" that means your level is above normal so you've recently had an

FACT:
A titer indicates whether the body has been fighting a particular infection by measuring antibodies to that infection in the blood.

infection. It takes a while for the immune system to produce enough antibodies to fight an infection. If you run a blood test on the same day you get sick, chances are you won't find an unusual level of antibodies. A few weeks later though, the titer will be elevated. Not every child with PANDAS will have an elevated or high strep titer, but most will. It also takes a while for the process to reverse itself, so the titer might stay elevated for quite some time.

Are There Different Antibodies? There are as many different types of antibodies as there are infections, so the physician needs to order the test specific for the infection. If a blood test is ordered for Lyme, the result will let you know if there are antibodies for Lyme in the bloodstream. But it will not, for example, pick up the presence of antibodies for strep, mononucleosis, hepatitis, or any other infection. Only a strep titer test will indicate whether you have produced antibodies to fight a strep infection.

What Is an Acquired Immunity? Acquired immunity is the body's memory system. Over time, our body often confronts the same bacteria. Each time, the body responds more effectively because our immune system remembers how to respond and does so more quickly. Vaccinations are based on the principle of acquired immunity. When we get a flu shot, we are injected with a bit of an invader virus and the body develops an immunity to it. If we are later exposed to the flu, because we have already produced the necessary antibodies once before, our bodies are already armed and ready to fight.

What Is a Compromised Immune System? There are two basic parts to a healthy immune system. The first is the ability to produce antibodies (think of it as manufacturing ammunition). The second is the ability to launch a targeted attack against only the invader and to stop when the job is done. A person has a compromised immune system when the body is not able to do one or both of those functions. Sometimes the compromise can be acquired through an infection that renders the immune system unable to function properly. Mononucleosis can do this on a temporary basis, and AIDS does so permanently. But other times, there is no clear explanation.

What Is an Autoimmune Disease? When the immune system turns on the body's healthy tissue and will not stop attacking, the patient has an autoimmune disease. A working immune system not only produces antibodies, but it is able to distinguish between the invaders and normal tissue. The antibodies launch a targeted attack. When the mission is accomplished, the immune system stops producing antibodies. A malfunctioning immune system may not perform either of these functions properly. It may become hyperactive and never stop producing antibodies, and it may also attack healthy tissue. Ordinarily antibodies lock only on the invasive or foreign antigens. But sometimes the antibodies goof up and lock onto tissues that have cell walls bearing a pattern similar to that of the invader. It's not a perfect fit, but it fits well enough. It's a case of mistaken identity. When the immune system makes antibodies to a foreign bacteria that then mistakenly attacks (or cross-reacts) with something similar to that invader, the medical term for what's happening is *molecular mimicry*.

> **FACT:**
> *An autoimmune disease is when the body's immune system misfires and attacks healthy cells.*

What Is Inflammation? Inflammation is another response of the immune system to infection. If you cut your finger, it becomes red and inflamed as the body rushes blood to the area. The blood is ready to produce antibodies that will fire on any invaders that may try to infect the cut. Without inflammation, the wound would never heal. When our body has a systemic infection, inflammation is everywhere, and immune chemicals call *cytokines* are likely out of whack. *Chronic inflammation* can lead to diseases such as hay fever, gum disease (periodontitis), and rheumatoid arthritis.

Infection and the Brain

How Do Infections and Antibodies Get into the Brain?
The *blood-brain barrier (BBB)* ordinarily keeps our brains insulated and safe. It is a tight network of capillaries that

> **FACT:**
> *The blood-brain barrier is what keeps our brains safe from most infections.*

prevent larger molecules such as bacteria, viruses, and antibodies from passing through to the brain. When we have the flu, we have aches and pains all over our body, but the brain stays safe because of that network. Things can change, though, if inflammation is persistent throughout the body. The capillaries expand and the blood-brain barrier becomes more permeable. When this happens, invaders and antibodies sometimes slip through the barrier and enter the brain. There are a few commonly known things that can cross the BBB even without inflammation: caffeine, nicotine, and psychotropic medication can all get through that tight network of capillaries and cross into the brain. *Psychotropic medicines* are those prescribed to address psychiatric conditions. Throughout this book the terms "psychotropic medication" and "psychiatric medication" are used interchangeably because they mean the same thing.

What Are the Basal Ganglia? The basal ganglia are a group of nuclei in the brain that act as a unit and control many behaviors and emotional functions. When the basal ganglia are disturbed, behavior is altered. Researchers believe the basal ganglia are under attack in PANDAS because so many of the children have the behavioral symptoms of tics and ADHD. Past research has shown that basal ganglia dysfunction is directly involved in those two disorders.

What Is a Neuropsychiatric Disorder? A neuropsychiatric disorder is one that occurs when mental disorders are related to disorders of the *nervous system*, which transmits signals through the different parts of our bodies. Therefore, a neuropsychiatric disorder involves both psychiatry (the treatment of mental disorders) and neurology (the treatment of disorders of the nervous system). Psychiatry and neurology were originally one branch of medicine, but became separate specialties about 100 years ago.

PANDAS

Now that we've covered the basics of infection and how the body responds, let's talk specifically about PANDAS. First you need to know that there are different kinds of strep and that strep is the abbreviation for Streptococci. Group A strep (GAS) causes sore throats and scarlet fever. Group B strep can cause serious problems for newborns when passed to them by their mothers during delivery. But PANDAS has only been linked to group A, so all references to "strep" throughout this book are to group A Streptococci. Strep is a powerful bacteria. It is one of the invaders that causes our bodies to need a helping hand, so antibiotics are routinely prescribed to treat it. Many of the physicians whose perspectives are presented in the appendix believe that childhood behavioral disorders may also be triggered by infections other than strep. They base this on their *clinical observations*, which are the things that doctors notice from treating patients. The things you notice as a parent are *anecdotal observations*. Clinical observations often lead to research studies, but strep is currently the only infection other than syphilis with a body of scientific research to support its link to a behavioral disorder. For that reason, this book primarily focuses on strep.

FACT: PANDAS is caused by the same bacteria that cause strep throat.

No body of medicine suddenly appears overnight. There is a long period of observation and attempted treatments that precede official recognition of the area, and an even longer time before the medical community agrees on an accepted treatment protocol. While the area is developing, individual doctors do their best to sort out the links between different illnesses and recoveries. PANDAS is no different than any other area of medicine. Its history includes a long chain of observations and treatment by trial and error. A line is often drawn between PANDAS and rheumatic fever because, at its essence, PANDAS is *rheumatic fever of the brain*.

What is rheumatic fever? Rheumatic fever occurs when strep antibodies attack the heart, usually about three weeks after strep throat. It is extremely serious, capable of causing permanent damage to the valves of the heart and sometimes death. It occurs more often in children than in adults. The reason that doctors prescribe antibiotics for strep is not to stop the sore throat; it's to prevent the patient from developing rheumatic fever.

How do we know strep causes rheumatic fever? During the 1940s, a series of studies on Navy servicemen demonstrated the correlation between strep and rheumatic fever. Every time there was an epidemic of scarlet fever (which is caused by strep), there would be an epidemic of rheumatic fever three weeks later. Once doctors started treating the scarlet fever with antibiotics, the rheumatic fever epidemics stopped. As a result of those studies, doctors then knew that strep had to be fully treated or rheumatic fever might develop. With the widespread availability of antibiotics following World War II, that is exactly what happened. As a result, rheumatic fever has been largely under control in the United States since the 1960s. There is no definitive test to diagnose rheumatic fever, so doctors do a careful exam, which includes listening to the heart, checking the joints, and ordering a strep titer blood test. Patients who develop rheumatic fever must remain on antibiotics for years.

☞

Many people have heard of rheumatic fever and have a general idea that it's heart damage resulting from a strep infection. Explaining PANDAS as "rheumatic fever of the brain" is sometimes a helpful analogy to use.

Why is rheumatic fever important to PANDAS? Rheumatic fever is similar to PANDAS because in both cases strep antibodies do the damage. In rheumatic fever, strep antibodies mistakenly attack healthy tissue in the heart. In PANDAS, strep antibodies attack the basal ganglia. A small number of patients who develop rheumatic fever also develop a movement disorder called Sydenham's chorea, and the movements of those patients helped lead to the identification PANDAS.

What is Sydenham's chorea? Sydenham's chorea (SC), which used to be called St. Vitus's Dance, shows up five to nine months after a strep infection. It affects more girls than boys. The patients who develop SC show emotional instability, muscle weakness, and quick, uncoordinated movements that are totally beyond their control. They flap their hands and jerk their arms. Their faces grimace. Their jaws stretch wide. These movements are called *chorea*, from the Latin word "dance."

How did Sydenham's chorea lead to identifying PANDAS? In the mid 1980s, researchers at the National Institute of Mental Health (NIMH) independently noticed that the movements of patients with chorea resembled the movements of patients with obsessive-compulsive disorder (OCD). About one-third of the children observed by the NIMH with OCD and tic disorders had choreiform movements. Because it was acknowledged that strep was the primary cause of the chorea movements, researchers wondered if strep might be at the root of OCD. Various studies were launched and a seminal paper was published in the *American*

FACT: Sydenham's chorea is a movement disorder associated with rheumatic fever, which is caused by strep.

Journal of Psychiatry in 1998. It was a study of 50 patients, and researchers reported a correlation between the presence of strep and OCD. It was called PANDAS. From that point on, although numerous studies have subsequently documented the correlation, a debate has raged in the medical community over PANDAS. This is not unusual in medicine. Breakthroughs almost always prompt controversy.

How can a strep infection cause a behavioral disorder? You've already learned several important PANDAS facts so far. They are:

- ❑ Our bodies produce antibodies when there is an infection.
- ❑ Antibodies sometimes mistakenly attack healthy tissue.
- ❑ Infection is accompanied by inflammation.
- ❑ Inflammation makes the blood-brain barrier (BBB) more permeable.
- ❑ The brain is less protected when the BBB is permeable.
- ❑ The basal ganglia of the brain control behavior.
- ❑ Strep antibodies can be vicious and attack the basal ganglia of the brain.

When strep antibodies pummel the area of the child's brain that controls behavior, the child's behavior changes. This does not happen to all children who have strep infections, just as not everyone with untreated strep will develop rheumatic fever. But the effect of strep antibodies on the brain may be overlooked and mistakenly excused to childhood misbehavior rather than recognized as symptomatic of the infection. Susan Swedo, MD, of the National Institute of Mental Health is one of the leading researchers in the country. She has reported studies showing that about 25 percent of first graders

FACT:

Two things happen when our bodies are fighting an infection: there is inflammation and the immune system produces antibodies.

have tics, particularly during the winter months when strep is most prevalent. And in collaboration with another of the country's top researchers, Tanya Murphy, MD, of the University of South Florida, she reported that all of those children who had classroom tics and behavioral problems tested positive for strep.

If a child has a strep infection, two things happen: inflammation develops and the immune system produces strep antibodies. With increased inflammation, the BBB may become more permeable. Swirling through our body's blood in pursuit of the strep, the antibodies cross the BBB and enter the brain. Once there, they form an imperfect lock with tissue in the basal ganglia that is mistaken for the strep bacteria; then the onslaught begins. At first the child may merely exhibit a mild tic or odd behavior. The children who are lucky enough to have traditional symptoms of strep may go to the pediatrician, turn up positive on a throat swab, take a ten-day course of antibiotics, and the whole thing subsides. The mild tics or behavioral outbursts are quickly forgotten.

The children who are not so lucky suffer because the strep is never detected or eradicated. As PANDAS progresses, the children may eventually be given mental health diagnoses such as OCD, ADHD, Tourette's, and/or bipolar disorder. They may be prescribed psychotropic medications, fall apart on a regular basis, and have difficulty functioning in a normal setting. Their heartbroken parents wonder what happened to their child and remember how he or she "used to be." The entire family revolves around the needs of the ill child. Siblings grow resentful, parents impatient, and the family structure teeters.

Parents who raise PANDAS as a possibility may be challenged by physicians who "don't believe" in PANDAS. Correct treatment may be further complicated by the information posted on the website for the National Institute of Mental Health. http://intramural.nimh.nih. gov/pdn/web.htm The criteria posted at the time of this writing are:

1. Presence of clinically significant obsessions, compulsion, and/or tics

2. Unusually abrupt onset of symptoms or a relapsing-remitting course of symptom severity
3. Prepubertal onset (with recognition that this is an arbitrary criteria chosen because post-strep reactions are rare after 12)
4. Association with other neuropsychiatric symptoms
5. Association with streptococcal infection

FACT:
Even if your child does not exactly fit the NIMH criteria, it doesn't mean your child does not have PANDAS. The criteria are simply guidelines.

Some doctors insist on strict compliance with the criteria. Keep in mind that my son had PANDAS, but he would not have fit the NIMH criteria. His symptoms developed over a period of weeks. He had no relapsing-remitting course of symptoms; he only grew consistently worse. And I had no way of associating his behaviors with a strep infection because we never knew he had one. He'd never had any traditional symptoms of strep, not even a sore throat. Moreover, as described by parents in the thousands of e-mails I have read, there are many other children who do not fit the NIMH criteria. They do, however, respond when appropriately treated for PANDAS.

What Is PANS? Also posted on the NIMH website is a suggested criteria for a disorder to be known as *PANS: Pediatric Acute-onset Neuropsychiatric Syndrome*. PANS was proposed by three researchers in early 2012 based on clinical observations made by treating physicians that bacteria and viruses other than strep can cause behavioral disorders. Although broader recognition of infectious triggers is a welcome change, the defined criteria for afflicted children is limiting. The threshold for fitting the criteria is a child who has OCD, which may manifest as "severely restricted food intake." If the threshold test is met by a child who has 1) OCD and/or an eating disorder, then 2) the child must have a severe and acute onset of at least two out of seven other specified concurrent

FACT:
If your child does not have OCD or an eating disorder, he does not fit the criteria for a disorder the NIMH calls PANS.

symptoms, and 3) there can be no better explanation for the behavioral disorder such as Sydenham's chorea, lupus, or Tourette's with the suggestion that spinal taps, EEGs, and MRIs may be appropriate to rule out these other possibilities.

The seven other neuropsychiatric symptoms specified by the NIMH for fulfilling part two of the PANS criteria are:

1. Anxiety (particularly, separation anxiety)
2. Emotional lability (extreme mood swings) and/or depression
3. Irritability, aggression, and/or severely oppositional behaviors
4. Behavioral (developmental) regression (examples, talking baby talk, throwing temper tantrums, etc)
5. Deterioration in school performance
6. Sensory or motor abnormalities
7. Somatic (bodily) signs and symptoms, including sleep disturbances, bedwetting, or urinary frequency

Parents are disappointed by the PANS criteria because the three-part rubric is so difficult for everyday pediatricians to apply. In particular, the children must be incredibly ill—essentially having reached a critical point and perhaps needing hospitalization—to be identified with PANS. Most acute PANS children do have a firestorm of these symptoms at onset and, therefore, an MRI, EEG, and LP are warranted. But many PANS children will not reach the acute stage if there is appropriate early intervention. And while most of the children do have OCD (perhaps manifesting as an eating problem), not all do. Some have only tics. For certain though, by the time a child has OCD, along with two out of the seven other behaviors, and a paper trail of diagnostic testing, that child will be unable to function. Not to mention that you will probably be broke. You are seeking intervention well before reaching that point. The PANS definition offers criteria to examine an extreme phenotype, but a solitary and new behavior in a previously asymptomatic child should be assessed

FACT:

An infectious trigger should be considered any time a child presents with a new behavior that interferes with daily life and is not consistent with the child's past behaviors.

for strep or other triggers. Early detection, immediate recognition, and prompt treatment are the keys to any neuropsychiatric disorder attributable to an infection.

SUMMING IT UP

Our brains are usually insulated because larger molecules such as bacteria, viruses, and antibodies cannot cross into the brain through a tight network of tiny blood vessels. The network that protects our brain is known as the blood-brain barrier. When there is inflammation due to an infection, the barrier becomes more permeable and molecules can enter the brain that ordinarily would not cross that barrier. When antibodies cross the blood-brain barrier they sometimes attack cells in the basal ganglia of the brain. This happens when the antibodies mistake healthy tissue for bacteria. Patients with antibodies misfiring on healthy tissue can display compulsions, obsessions, tics, and a whole host of other behaviors that may indicate PANDAS. For these patients, behavioral disorders and sometimes psychiatric diagnoses may indicate that the true problem is an infection.

BIG IDEAS FROM CHAPTER TWO

❑ Pathogens are bacteria or viruses that cause infections.
❑ The immune system produces antibodies or "war troops" that are specific to each infection.
❑ A titer test detects a particular infection through blood work by measuring the antibodies to that specific infection.
❑ Over time, the immune system will respond more quickly to an infection that it recognizes.
❑ A compromised immune system does not successfully fight an infection.
❑ An autoimmune disease occurs when a patient's immune system attacks healthy tissue.
❑ Inflammation is a response to infection.
❑ The blood-brain barrier (BBB) insulates the brain from infection, but can become permeable to pathogens and antibodies with inflammation.   *(continued)*

- ❑ The basal ganglia of the brain act as a unit to control behaviors.
- ❑ Group A Streptococci are powerful bacteria, and our bodies often need the help of antibiotics to fight off strep.
- ❑ OCD, tics and/or difficult behaviors may indicate the presence of strep or other infections.
- ❑ Children who do not exactly fit within the NIMH criteria may still have an infection as the root cause of their behavioral difficulties.
- ❑ A solitary and new behavior in a previously asymptomatic child should be assessed for strep or other triggers.

How Is the Condition Diagnosed?

3

Dear Beth,

My daughter is almost eight years old, and I believe she has PANDAS. I have been taking her to see a therapist for the past two weeks who diagnosed her with OCD. She never had any signs of OCD until she was sick with strep throat in January, and she's never been the same. She was a model student with good grades. Now she can't focus and her "crazy brain" keeps racing with crazy thoughts. She is depressed, often cries at the drop of a hat, and it's difficult to calm her back down. She is really struggling and has even written me a note asking for a new life and praying to God to take this away from her and make her normal again. I need some help! Can you tell me any doctors who can help me? We are seeing her pediatrician tomorrow, but she has no clue! Thank God I found this info myself!

Hoping to Hear

Could It Be PANDAS?

There is no conclusive test to determine whether a child has PANDAS. It's a clinical diagnosis, meaning that a knowledgeable doctor will take a full history and then piece together various threads of information to determine whether your child has the disorder. The doctor will want to consider a description of your child's behaviors, when and how they started, any mental health diagnoses, the child's response to prior psychiatric medications, your child's history of infections and response to antibiotics, the results of swabs, cultures, and blood tests, your family's medical history, and the doctor's own personal observation of the child. It takes a patient, careful, open-minded

What the doctor says:

"The onus is on physicians to do a careful clinical inquiry, which means digging into the child's pediatric medical records. When were the throat cultures done? What did they show? What antibiotics were prescribed and taken over what period of time? What was the response?"

Daniel Geller, MD
Massachusetts General Hospital, Boston

physician to determine whether a child has PANDAS. This chapter is about what happens along the way toward reaching a diagnosis of PANDAS, or deciding that it might be something else.

The Mental Health Evaluation

Most children who visit a PANDAS doctor already have a mental health diagnosis. You know from reading the earlier chapters that it might be OCD, a tic disorder, ADHD, separation anxiety, Tourette's disorder, and/or a host of other psychiatric illnesses. Often those diagnoses will be determined through a mental health evaluation following a referral made by your pediatrician or family doctor. Sometimes schools may suggest an evaluation if the child's classroom behaviors are concerning. Evaluations are often made by doctorate-level psychologists who may specialize in diagnosing conditions, but not offer treatment. Other times, the evaluation will be made by a psychiatrist. At the conclusion of the evaluation, the diagnosis will be made.

Regardless of how your child arrived at the point of being evaluated (unless it is the result of a crisis hospitalization), a thorough evaluation will cover the same basic steps. You will be asked to fill out questionnaires about your family history. School records and observations will be supplied. Various tests will be administered. Behavioral charts and reports will be reviewed. The child and/or caregivers will participate in interviews. The process will most likely involve several visits.

When the diagnosis is made, it will be rendered based upon the *Diagnostic and Statistical Manual of Mental Disorders*, otherwise known as the *DSM*. The *DSM* is published by the American Psychiatric Association and the goal is nationwide consistency. By following the criteria set forth in the *DSM*, what a practitioner diagnoses as OCD in New York should also be diagnosed as OCD in California. The *DSM* was first published in 1952 and is now in its 5th Edition (*DSM*-5). An infection subtype was proposed for the *DSM*-5, but did not make it into the edition.

> **FACT:**
> *The DSM sets forth the criteria for mental health disorders to provide nationwide diagnostic consistency. PANDAS is not listed in the DSM.*

If your child's behaviors are severe by the time of the evaluation, he may already be taking psychotropic medication under the care of a physician. Even when children are diagnosed in a hospital and released with medication, the caregiver is instructed to follow up with another doctor. Ideally, the child should see a developmental pediatrician or a child psychiatrist for follow-up. But due to the difficulty of obtaining an appointment with one of those specialists (because there are so few of them), it is becoming increasingly common for pediatricians to take the lead in prescribing psychotropic medications.

By the time you are reading this book, all or some of the individuals mentioned above may already be involved in your child's life. Perhaps your child has a diagnosis, and he is on medication. At some point, though, you started wondering if the diagnosis was correct, and you started asking questions.

There are two stumbling blocks along the way to considering PANDAS. First, PANDAS is not in the *DSM* so it's tough to find practitioners who have the expertise to diagnose, much less treat, the disorder. Second, mental health evaluations for children usually do not include physical health as a component. Therefore, it's doubtful that the presence of an infection will be considered unless you bring it up.

There are exceptions. There are some treatment providers who are alert to PANDAS. When the child comes into their office with an onset of concerning behaviors, those providers immediately consider whether the symptoms may indicate an infection. Savvy practitioners might ask whether there is a family history of autoimmune disease. They might also look for the clusters of symptoms that may further indicate the presence of PANDAS: separation anxiety with nighttime

What the doctor says:

"PANDAS may present primarily as OCD and/or tics,
but it will often be accompanied by other symptoms.
Uncontrollable movements, separation anxiety, enuresis,
getting 'stuck ' in an OCD way are all red flags for
me. And I find that children who have true Tourette's
generally do not have the other symptoms such as anxiety
or enuresis."

Catherine Nicolaides, MD
Children's Specialized Hospital
Egg Harbor, NJ

fears and enuresis/daytime urinary frequency, ADHD with emotional lability and cognitive changes, and motoric symptoms—tics and motoric hyperactivity, simple compulsive rituals, and handwriting changes. But not all doctors have the knowledge that will cause them to explore those areas.

Making the Diagnosis

Because so many of you will be looking for the signs yourself, it will be helpful to understand how PANDAS doctors generally diagnose the disorder. Keep in mind that medicine is not an exact science so no description can be all inclusive. There will always be variations and exceptions, particularly with a disorder that is relatively "new." For more specific treatment approaches, you will want to read each of the interviews presented in the appendix. In general, PANDAS doctors are looking for behavioral onsets or exacerbations that are not consistent with past history and can be linked to an infection.

I am going to use my son's case as an example because, in retrospect, it should have been "easy" to diagnose. Why should it have been easy to spot? Because he had *three classic hallmarks* of the disorder.

1. Rapid Behavioral Deterioration. Sammy had eleven solid years of functional behavior. Shortly after his twelfth birthday, he went from baseline to completely dysfunctional in a period of six weeks. At the end of those six weeks, he literally could not get out the front door. While he grew progressively worse, we visited a doctorate-level psychologist. After a number of sessions with the psychologist, he recommended that we see a child psychiatrist for a "rule out" of OCD. Treatment providers use the term "rule out" when they suspect a disorder. If they are thinking about OCD, they don't say, "Let's see if he has OCD," or, "I think he has OCD." They say, "We need a rule out on OCD." The fact that my formerly "normal" child rapidly descended into a behavioral disorder was a sign that he had PANDAS.

2. Failure to Respond to Typical Treatments. The psychologist gave me a list of names of child psychiatrists, and I began calling. It was quite an effort to get an appointment within a reasonable timeframe. At our first appointment, the child psychiatrist diagnosed Sammy with OCD. The diagnosis was made based on the list of behaviors in which he was engaging. He was prescribed a selective serotonin reuptake inhibitor, an SSRI. As is typical of the introduction of psychotropic medications, Sammy started at a small dose that gradually increased. Over the course of a year, despite the ever increasing dosage, he never got better. He only got worse, even with all the behavioral counseling sessions he attended. In retrospect, the fact that Sammy never responded to the prescribed medication and counseling, which are the typical treatments, was a sign that he had PANDAS.

> **FACT:**
> *Three classic hallmarks of PANDAS are:*
> - *rapid deterioration*
> - *failure to respond to typical treatments*
> - *positive for strep*

3. Positive for Strep. By word of mouth I learned, as so many of you have, that my child's mental health disorder might be attributable to strep. The next piece made it "easy" for us, the results of his blood tests. Although to the best of my knowledge he'd never had strep, blood work turned up positive for strep and showed an elevated titer (high level of antibodies) for the infection. When a patient has a strep infection without the classic symptoms—no sore throat, temperature, and so forth—the patient is *asymptomatic*. Although Sammy was asymptomatic for strep, he had an elevated titer. Not every PANDAS child has an elevated strep titer, but mine did. Coupled with his rapid deterioration and failure to respond to the SSRIs, his elevated titer was another sign that he had PANDAS.

Detecting the Infection

> ## What the doctor says:
>
> *"My advice is listen to what the parents are saying. When parents say their child is so dramatically different, that this is not like their child, those would be clues to do an infection work up."*
>
> Tanya Murphy, MD

Grade schools are petri dishes for strep. They are full of adorable little children not washing their hands, sneezing into the air, and wiping their noses in many places other than tissues. As a result, strep is rampant in grade schools. Strep does not have to be in the throat. For example, it can also be present in the tonsils, the intestinal tract (or "gut"), and the anus. It is not so important to know where the infection resides: what matters is to know it is present. There are three ways to detect a strep infection: a rapid strep test, a culture, and a blood test. Both the rapid strep test and the culture require a throat swab.

Rapid Strep Tests and Cultures: Your situation is one of the easier ones if your child has a documented history of strep. You may be able to correlate the onset or exacerbation of your child's behaviors with a strep throat. If you suspect PANDAS, there are preliminary steps you will most likely take before running blood work. The first step will be a rapid strep test. Some doctors are reluctant to swab the child when she does not have a sore throat or a temperature, so you may have to be quite insistent. A few parents have reported that doctors tried to appease them by taking a quick look at the throat and announcing, "It's not strep." There is no research supporting a doctor's ability to 100 percent diagnose strep simply by looking, so stay firm and insist on a swab. As you continue to press, you may find yourself in somewhat of a battle by insisting that your child be tested. Ultimately, if your child turns up positive, your doctor may be stunned by the result and perhaps be transformed into a believer. But if the test turns up negative, don't give up.

A rapid strep test is a highly effective gauge of a current strep-infected throat when it is properly administered, but that often isn't what happens. To be effective, the sample has to be swabbed from the back of the throat. When properly administered, the swabbing will often cause the child to gag. Health-care providers would prefer not to cause children to gag, so many times the test is not properly performed. The result will then be a false negative. If you suspect PANDAS and the rapid strep test is negative, you must next ask for a throat culture. A culture is somewhat more reliable because the bacteria is given the opportunity to grow overnight. Again, your provider may be resistant, but stay insistent and clear. There are many parents whose children had negative rapid strep tests, but turned up positive on a throat culture.

Blood Work: Finally, while swabs and cultures let you know if there is a current infection in the throat, they do not detect older infections or when strep is elsewhere in the body. The definitive way to find evidence of a strep infection is by searching for strep antibodies in the blood. Even if your child has a positive swab or culture, you will want to begin tracking antibodies through the blood. Make sure your child drinks plenty of water about an hour before the blood test because that will help the blood to be drawn much easier. It is painful for everyone involved when blood must be drawn from a dehydrated child.

FACT:
There are three ways to detect strep:
1. Rapid strep test*
2. Culture*
3. Blood Test

*Both of these involve throat swabs.

☞
Have your child drink a glass or two of water about an hour before a blood test. It will help the blood draw go more smoothly.

FACT:
There are two blood tests for strep: ASO and Anti-DNase B.

There are two blood tests that detect whether there are strep antibodies in the system. One is an *ASO titer test*, and the other is for *Anti-DNase B*. ASO stands for Antistreptolysin O. Anti-DNase B stands for Anti-deoxyribonuclease B. Streptolysin O and Deoxyriboneclease-B are both substances produced by strep bacteria. The tests measure the antibodies that the immune system has produced to fight the strep bacteria. The results of these tests should be available within 24 to 48 hours.

An ASO test will come back positive or negative. If your child ever had strep at any point in his life, it may still be positive. This is because once a person contracts strep, some level of antibodies for Streptolysin O will remain in the system. When Sammy's test came back positive, I was shocked because as far as I knew he'd never had strep.

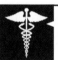

What the doctor says:

"I now check ASO titers in every new patient who has any kind of repetitive behavior or possible compulsion."

Richard Livingston, MD
Vista Health Services
Ft. Smith, Arkansas

A titer is the measure of the concentration of antibodies in the blood. What's important is whether the titer is elevated. If the titer is elevated, it means your child had a strep infection in the recent past. The Anti-DNase B test also reports a titer. A word of caution: specifically point out to the lab that your prescription is for an Anti-DNase B test and *not* for an Anti-DNA test. If the lab assistant incorrectly enters the order, you'll end up with the results of an Anti-DNA test, which is totally different and useless for PANDAS. I learned this the hard way. After waiting for days, when I finally got the result, I realized that the lab had run the wrong test. After that, the wrong lab was run again only once and that was the one other time when I forgot to remind the lab assistant to run the correct test. The lab isn't always happy to hear you making your expectation

*Make sure the lab runs a test for Anti-DNase B, **not** an Anti-DNA test.*

clear, but take a deep breath and state what you need. This is your child's health, and they need to get it right.

Reading a blood test: As the CEO of your child's life, you should obtain physical copies of the blood test results. Some results will be positive or negative. Other results will report a number. For any blood test that is ordered (not just strep), there is a number or range that is considered normal. When a test comes back with a number that is abnormal, it will usually be flagged. In fact, there is often a column that says, "FLAG." Some labs do not flag abnormal results, but you can usually figure it out by reading the number or range that is considered normal. If your child's number falls within the range, then the result is normal. Outside the range is abnormal.

There may be variations in standards set by different labs, but ordinarily an ASO titer under 200 is considered normal. If you ran my blood for strep today, my ASO would come back POS (positive) with a titer of 100. This is because I have had strep infections in my life, but I have not had one for quite some time. My titer is low. Sammy's test came back POS with a titer of 800. His titer was elevated. Most—but not all—PANDAS children will have an elevated titer.

Titers need to be adjusted for age. Among children, preschoolers have lower positive titers, and seven to twelve year olds have the highest. So if age adjusted, an ASO of 150 may be positive for a five-year-old, but negative for an eight-year-old. Therefore, a preschooler with sudden behaviors and an ASO titer under 200 warrants careful consideration. Keep in mind that titers are estimated to follow a strep infection by four to six weeks. Therefore, you might get a positive throat swab, but a normal titer because it takes time for the titer to rise. A positive swab with a normal titer most likely means there is a current infection, but the immune system has not yet fully kicked in. If you run the blood a month or so later, you will most likely see an elevation. The most definitive test for recent strep is a titer that doubles when tested at onset and then four to six weeks later.

Of course this set of facts will not be the norm for every child. Some children have compromised immune systems that do not produce antibodies to the infection. Some children have elevated titers with no behaviors. Once a child has suffered a PANDAS episode, it appears that subsequent infections such as mycoplasma, Lyme, and the flu can all trigger behaviors. At this time, however, strep is the only bacteria other than syphilis with research supporting the link between the infection and a mental health disorder.

Precautions to Take with Strep

A PANDAS child will continue to have behavioral exacerbations when exposed to strep, so it's important to do the best you can to eliminate the possibility of reinfection. First and foremost, you must consider whether others in the home might have the bacteria. It is crucial that everyone in the house be tested for strep and, if need be, treated. Asymptomatic family members may be strep carriers who are reinfecting the PANDAS child. Carriers may require a combination of antibiotics to eliminate the infection.

Test all household members for strep, including the family dog.

When testing for carriers, don't forget the family dog. Often overlooked, the dog can be the reason that strep is a recurrent problem in your home. While a dog will not show symptoms of strep, it can be a carrier. Strep in a dog is detected through a culture. The veterinarian will need to sedate the dog because it's important that the swab be taken from far back in the throat. The culture is then sent to the lab. For a dog carrying strep, the veterinarian will prescribe Clavamox (which is essentially Augmentin) in a dosage appropriate for the dog's weight. Given the complexity and expense of testing a dog for strep, you might ask if the veterinarian is simply willing to assume that the dog has strep and prescribe the Clavamox.

Become a strep vigilante: regularly scrub the bathrooms and kitchen, change the toothbrushes, wash the sheets and towels.

Next, focus on your home. Replace all the toothbrushes, wash the sheets and towels, scrub all bathrooms, and wipe down the kitchen. Discourage siblings from sharing toothbrushes and towels. And ask your child's teacher to let you know when there is a strep outbreak at school. Your child cannot live in a bubble, but you can do your best to make your child's environment as safe as possible and to be alert to the existence of possible triggers.

SUMMING IT UP

It is wise to consider whether an underlying infection might be a cause of your child's behaviors, but there is no definitive test for PANDAS and it is not yet described in the *Diagnostic and Statistical Manual of Mental Disorders (DSM-5)*. A PANDAS diagnosis requires careful consideration of a number of factors that will be culled from a complete medical history. Not every disorder can be attributed to an infection, but PANDAS must be considered if your child has had rapidly deteriorating behaviors, failed to respond to psychiatric medication, and has tested positive for strep. If you believe strep is the culprit, you must make certain it is eliminated from your household by testing all family members (including the family dog) and doing a thorough cleaning.

BIG IDEAS FROM CHAPTER THREE

❑ PANDAS is a clinical diagnosis; there is no definitive test.
❑ PANDAS is not in the mental health reference manual called the *DSM*, which stands for *Diagnostic and Statistical Manual of Mental Disorders*.
❑ Three classic hallmarks of PANDAS are:
  Rapid deterioration
  Failure to respond to typical treatments of psychotropic medication and behavioral intervention
  Positive for strep infection (and possibly other infections as well).
❑ Strep can be asymptomatic: no sore throat or fever.
❑ There are three ways to detect strep:
  a rapid throat swab
  a throat culture
  two blood tests: ASO and Anti-DNase B.
❑ Your child needs to drink plenty of water at least one hour before a blood test.
❑ Check the blood test results for "flags," or numbers that do not fall within the stated normal range.
❑ Titers, which measure antibodies, lag behind the infection by four to six weeks.
❑ If you have or suspect a PANDAS child, test every household member for strep, including the family dog.

II   MANAGING THE DISORDER

Medical Treatment

Dear Beth,

Our daughter who is ten was diagnosed with strep throat in January of this year. Almost immediately I watched the life in my daughter's eyes disappear as she was overcome with separation anxiety...horrible repetitive thoughts that now ran her day...constant crying in school... germ phobias that made her daily life impossible...I knew all along that something was terribly wrong and when I Googled for help your site came up and described my once-vibrant child to a T....How should we get started with treatment?

Thank You,
A Very Concerned and Thankful Parent

How Is It Treated?

One of the tough things about PANDAS is that there is no consensus about the best way to treat it. There is, however, agreement on the four goals of a comprehensive treatment plan:

❑ Manage the infection
❑ Reduce inflammation and build the immune system
❑ Address the psychiatric symptoms
❑ Help the child develop the skills needed to manage his behaviors during recovery

Each physician will approach these goals differently and achieving some of these goals requires medication. Others require behavioral and dietary intervention. For those who recognized PANDAS early, an aggressive pediatrician may be all you need. Other children will need multiple providers as outlined in chapter 7, "Assembling the Treatment Team of Doctors and Other Clinicians." Regardless of the course you follow, PANDAS requires patience and persistence because treating any mental health disorder is a trial and error process. By understanding the various treatment choices, you will be able to make informed decisions about which approach is best for your child.

This chapter will outline the current treatment approaches and direct you to other sections of this book as needed. At the end of this chapter is a description of one boy's experience with IV Ig, so that if you choose that route you will be familiar with what to expect with that procedure.

The appendix at the end of this book contains the full text of comprehensive interviews with a number of treating physicians. Those interviews contain a wealth of information, and you will want to review them for even more detail on treatments.

Manage the Infection

What the doctor says:

"My 'go-to' treatment is one of the cillins: amoxicillin or Augmentin seems to work best."

Richard Livingston, MD

Any mental health disorder is difficult to treat, even when it is not attributed to a current infection. For example, providing the schizophrenic brain with what it needs to function normally becomes a lifelong challenge for the afflicted and their doctors. The good news about PANDAS, though, is that with proper treatment it does not need to be a lifelong disorder. PANDAS usually manifests when the patients are children. With early and appropriate intervention, it does not appear to cause permanent damage, possibly because the brain continues to develop throughout childhood.

FACT:
PANDAS does not have to be a lifelong disorder.

You know from reading chapter 1 that PANDAS is believed to be caused by strep antibodies entering the brain. Therefore, the first goal of treating a PANDAS child is to knock out the infection that

What the doctor says:

"I work closely with an ENT. If the patient has sleep issues or adenoid problems, the ENT may recommend removal of the tonsils or adenoids."

Eric Hollander, MD,
Mondefiore Medical Center

is triggering the production of antibodies. There are three ways that physicians address the infection:

❑ antibiotics
❑ tonsillectomies
❑ blood procedures

What can be unclear is where in the body the infection resides. It may be in the throat, but other possibilities include the sinuses and tonsils, the gut, and the area around the anus. When group A strep shows up in the area around the anus, which is called *perianal strep*, it is often confused for diaper rash in very young children.

1. Antibiotics. The first line of treatment for any serious bacterial infection will always be antibiotics. If effective, that will be the simplest method of treating the infection causing PANDAS. One problem is that often the doctor will order the typical prescription and that will not be of sufficient strength or duration for PANDAS. This is not an ordinary strep infection that will respond nicely to a ten-day course of the recommended dose of penicillin. Treatment has to be aggressive. Therefore, the questions are:

❑ Which antibiotic is the right one to prescribe?
❑ What is the correct dose?
❑ How long should your child take it?

These are questions your doctors must ultimately answer, but here is some basic background. Different antibiotics work differently. Some prevent a cell wall from forming. Others stop the bacteria from multiplying. But what they all aim to do is kill the bacteria causing the infection. When the infection is strep, doctors will routinely prescribe penicillin-based antibiotics: penicillin itself, amoxicillin or Augmentin. Penicillin-based antibiotics are the antibiotics of choice for two reasons. First, there is no indication that strep develops a resistance to penicillin. Second, while penicillin is highly effective against strep, it is not particularly effective against much else other than syphilis.

Other antibiotics, such as azithromycin or clarithromycin, are called broad spectrum antibiotics because they are effective against a number of different bacteria. Broad spectrum antibiotics have "better eradication"; they will go after almost whatever bacteria may be present. In fact, when there is an infection and a doctor is not quite sure what it might be, a broad spectrum antibiotic such as azithromycin may be prescribed. The concern about treating strep with a broad spectrum antibiotic is that the strep might develop a resistance and inadvertently become a super-bug. For that reason, many doctors feel that avoiding a broad spectrum antibiotic whenever possible is generally prudent; others feel that is what results in the best response in some cases of PANDAS.

If you are using a liquid antibiotic, make sure it is always fresh. A liquid antibiotic is reconstituted by mixing the powder with water, and it loses its effectiveness after ten days.

Of course, when a patient is allergic to penicillin, then the doctor will have no choice but to prescribe a different antibiotic. And some doctors have found that the bacteria causing the behaviors is not strep.

What the doctor says:

"My first choice is Augmentin when the presentation is tics. For acute, severe OCD presentations, I prescribe azithromycin, and I've found mycoplasma in many of those cases. I start with the standard dose."

Tanya Murphy, MD

Once the child stabilizes and remains stable for at least a couple of months on the medication, many doctors feel that the best approach is to try weaning the antibiotics to see what happens. Stopping "cold turkey" may throw a child into an exacerbation. And with each exacerbation the symptoms grow worse. With patience, you and your doctor will be able to find out whether your child is ready to maintain on a lesser dose of antibiotics and when she can be weaned completely. Be advised that there are some children who must remain on antibiotics for years; Sammy was one of them.

What the doctor says:

"I believe that for purposes of this disorder, the antibiotic should be titrated (gradually increased) and withdrawn similarly to psychotropic medication."

Catherine Nicolaides, MD

When your child takes an extended course of any antibiotic, it is also important for him to take probiotics. This is because antibiotics will wipe out all bacteria in the intestine: good and bad. We need good bacteria to help digest food. Without good bacteria the intestinal tract is out of balance. This can lead to something called "leaky gut syndrome," which is discussed in more detail in chapter 6, "Nutritional Considerations." For now, just remember that it's best to supplement your child's diet with probiotics when taking long-term antibiotics.

Remember to give your child probiotics when she is taking long- term antibiotics, and not at the same time as she takes the antibiotic.

And the probiotics should not be taken at the same time as the antibiotic or each will be less effective. For example, if your child is taking antibiotics with breakfast, have him take his probiotics with dinner.

2. Tonsillectomy. The tonsils are a prime area of the body for harboring strep. There is a split among physicians on whether surgically removing these organs will be helpful. The job of the tonsils is to catch bacteria that try to enter through the mouth. Tonsillitis occurs when the tonsils become inflamed and infected. If the infection does not respond to antibiotics, tonsils are sometimes removed. Tonsillectomies used to be performed fairly frequently, but medical practice has changed and now the procedure is not so prevalent. Some parents are certain that a tonsillectomy is what caused their child to finally start getting better. Other parents report results ranging from moderate improvement to none at all, and sometimes an exacerbation following the procedure. The theory that a tonsillectomy will help stems from the fact that strep can hide in the tonsils. Studies have reported that children with recurrent strep throat benefit from tonsillectomies, but as of this writing there has not been any research that specifically studies tonsillectomies and PANDAS patients.

3. Blood Procedures. The other way that PANDAS is sometimes treated is with a blood procedure. There are two: one is called *plasmapheresis* and the other is *intravenous immunoglobulin (IV Ig)*.

Plasmapheresis is a procedure whereby blood is removed from the body and essentially cleansed of antibodies before being returned to the body. Plasmapheresis is used to treat immune disorders such as lupus

What the doctor says:

"A tonsillectomy is a bloody operation and handling that tissue, potentially laden with strep, can cause the bacteria to disburse throughout the system, resulting in a post-op behavioral exacerbation. For that reason, ten days before a tonsillectomy, I start the patient on clindamycin in an effort to sterilize the tonsil tissue before surgical removal."

Rosario Trifiletti, MD
Pediatric Neurologist, Ramsey, NJ

and Guillain-Barré syndrome. On occasion, it is used to treat PANDAS patients, but those occasions are extremely rare. Plasmapheresis for PANDAS patients is usually preceded by a demonstrated failure to respond to IV Ig.

IV Ig is the infusion of a pooled blood product into the patient's body, which contains IgG (antibodies) extracted from the blood of thousands of donors. Most people know what an IV looks like. It is a bag of liquid solution that hangs from a tall metal pole. The solution drips through a thin plastic line that runs from the bag to a needle that has been inserted into the patient's vein. IV Ig can be administered in a doctor's office, in a hospital, or at an infusion center. Sometimes the infusion can take place at the patient's home. When a patient is receiving medication through an IV, the patient must remain connected to the bag of solution for the duration of the treatment unless a professional disconnects the line.

IV Ig is administered for a variety of reasons to patients with autoimmune diseases. It can help counter autoimmune reactions by introducing different antibodies into the system and perhaps by targeting the cells that are producing the dangerous antibodies. Because IV Ig is collected from many donors, it may also supply a sick child with antibodies that child is missing. IV Ig is rarely a "one stop" solution; it is routinely repeated in treating other medical conditions and that is also true for PANDAS patients. The effects

What the doctor says:

"I urge caution about the use of IV Ig because the children relapse with only one treatment. I've observed that some children do better after three treatments, but they have by no means remitted. My feeling is that IV Ig is not appropriate unless the children can be defined as immune deficient or there is otherwise biological evidence that warrants the treatment. I am more open to it, however, for children who do not respond to antibiotics."

Tanya Murphy, MD

are generally believed to last up to three months. For PANDAS, IV Ig must be coupled with antibiotics. Without sufficient antibiotic treatment, the children rarely achieve lasting behavioral gains.

One reason behaviors improve after IV Ig is that the infusion is also believed to help reduce inflammation and thus to close the blood-brain barrier (BBB). This temporarily helps to prevent additional antibodies from crossing to enter the brain. The antibodies that are already in the brain degenerate over time, which is why the child's behaviors begin to diminish. But IV Ig does not address the underlying infection; it only addresses the antibodies that the body produces in response to the infection. If the infection is not treated, or if the child is exposed again, more antibodies will be produced, inflammation will return, the BBB becomes permeable, antibodies will flow in to the brain, and the cycle begins again. Typically, at that point, the IV Ig treatment will be repeated.

FACT:
In 2011 the American Red Cross and the CDC identified two potential risks associated with the blood supply.

The risks associated with introducing a pooled blood product into your child's system must be carefully weighed. There are some children who will not respond to antibiotics. For those children, IV Ig and perhaps even plasmapheresis may be the only option. But taking one of those steps without first determining whether your child will respond to sufficient, long-term antibiotics may be premature. We are always told the blood supply is safe, but it's safe only from what we know to look for. The blood supply was "safe" when soldiers serving in Vietnam contracted Hepatitis C from IV Ig infusions. It was also "safe" when the AIDS virus was transmitted through tainted blood. In 2011, the American Red Cross stopped taking blood from donors with a history of chronic fatigue syndrome due to concerns about a possible viral connection. During that same year, the CDC issued a press release stating that Babesia, a tick-borne parasite of red blood cells, is in the blood supply.

Another factor to weigh about IV Ig is the cost. It's prohibitive, averaging roughly $100 per pound of the child's weight. So IV Ig for a one hundred pound child will cost $10,000, and it is not always covered by insurance.

What the doctor says:

"Ninety percent of the time, PANDAS/PANS can be treated with antibiotics and mild anti-inflammatories without the need for IV Ig or plasmapheresis."

Rosario Trifiletti, MD

Reduce Inflammation and Build the Immune System

The reason you want to reduce inflammation is to help seal the blood-brain barrier (BBB) so that strep antibodies will not cross into the brain. You also want to build your child's immune system so that it can effectively battle infections. Both these goals can be helped by taking the dietary steps covered in chapter 6, "Nutritional Considerations."

What the doctor says:

"My approach is two fold: address the immune dysfunction and treat the infection."

Dr. Ali Carine
Integrative Osteopathic Pediatrician
Columbus, OH

Medically, there are two possible approaches to reducing inflammation:

- ❑ ibuprofen
- ❑ steroids

The first and easiest may be to try giving your child ibuprofen. As an anti-inflammatory, parents have found that it sometimes helps "take the edge off." It's by no means a cure, but it may help. This approach warrants caution, however, as more concerns are being raised that it may be "nephrotoxic," meaning to cause liver damage.

Second, sometimes doctors will prescribe a short course of steroids to see if behaviors improve. These are not the same class of steroids as those taken by athletes, but rather those prescribed to help reduce inflammation. Prednisone or cortisone are examples of steroids typically prescribed to help with inflammatory conditions such as asthma and arthritis. If the child's behaviors improve with steroids, the prescribing physician may feel this is further evidence that the child has PANDAS. The theory is that the anti-inflammatory effect of the steroid is helping to seal the BBB and, therefore, fewer antibodies reaching the brain result in less behaviors. Not all patients respond well to steroids, though, and the side effects can be concerning. Some patients become aggressive, agitated, and out of control. If your child is on steroids and you see those sorts of behaviors, get in touch with your doctor right away. Steroids are never prescribed long term.

FACT:
A "steroid burst" is a course of steroids given in high doses for a few days.

What the doctor says:

"Steroids can only be prescribed short term. For a long-term natural anti-inflammatory, I recommend a high dose of fish oil—2000 mg to 3000 mg per day—of Omega 3 fats. Another natural anti-inflammatory is the Indian spice Turmeric. The active ingredient in Turmeric is Curcumin. For this I recommend a supplement called Enhansa to my patients."

Robert Sears, MD, FAAP (Dr. Bob)
Capistrano Beach, California

Address the Psychiatric Symptoms

Psychotropic medicine is prescribed to help change the chemistry of the brain so that behaviors are modified while the infection is addressed. Effectively prescribing psychotropic medication requires not only thorough familiarity with the various medications, but great skill, persistence, and patience. Psychiatrists

What the doctor says:

"I will prescribe traditional psychotropic medication to address the psychiatric symptoms as needed, but generally not concurrently with antibiotics. I want to allow the antibiotics a chance to work before committing a child to a course of psychotropic medication."

Daniel Geller, MD

and developmental pediatricians are specifically trained in this area of medicine.

Working with psychotropic medication is a delicate balance because it must be adjusted based upon the patient's response. The prescription always starts at a low dose and then gradually increases—to the maximum recommended dose—until the desired behavioral effect is achieved. For example, if your child is experiencing extreme anxiety, the prescription will be increased until the anxiety lessens. The maximum recommended dose is based on the child's weight. When first introduced, the body is slow to process the medication. As the body adjusts and begins to process the medication more quickly, the dosage must be increased to achieve the desired response. There will be increases and decreases over time to reach the right balance. Sometimes, patients stop responding to a particular medication that was formerly effective. If that happens, the doctor will need to prescribe something different.

You are the observer who is best able to judge what is going on with the prescribed medication, so accurately monitoring your child's response is crucial. Equally

FACT:
"Titrating" psychotropic medication means gradually increasing the amount until you reach the correct therapeutic dose; that means achieving the desired behavioral response and not exceeding the manufacturer's recommended limits.

important is your ability to clearly convey that information to the doctor. Doctors can only work with the information they are given. If it's not accurate, or if they have to sort through extraneous information to understand what is going on, the process will slow. As Observer in Chief, you need to know the name of what your child is taking, when she takes it, the desired effect it should produce, whether you are seeing that result or something else, and the potential side effects to watch for.

Help with Behavioral Skills

Children with PANDAS don't just wake up one day without behaviors as a result of taking medication. They need help developing the skills that will conquer those behaviors and that usually means cognitive behavioral therapy (CBT). Through CBT, the children learn to overcome the behaviors that have come to define them. First though, the child must be well enough to participate in the therapy. If you try to introduce it too early, CBT will not be effective. The extent of the therapy will usually depend upon how long the child has had PANDAS and how ingrained the behaviors have become. Some children who are highly motivated and determined will be able to work with a psychologist once a week and then practice the skills at home. Other children are so dominated by behaviors that they may need to enter a residential program for more intensive work. Behavioral therapy is so important to recovery that chapter 5, "Cognitive Behavioral Therapy" is devoted exclusively to this topic.

An IV Ig Story

Keith was eleven when he needed IV Ig. He had a history of increasing aggression with a clear pattern of strep and other infections. His PANDAS treatment was complicated due to a penicillin allergy and, although he was treated with different antibiotics, he never responded well and could not attend school. Eventually, IV Ig was prescribed by his out-of-state pediatric neurologist, and he responded well to his first treatment. Keith's mom said he was "80 percent back" within six weeks, but after six months the behaviors began to return. His grades fell, he would spin in his chair at school, and he became more aggressive with his classmates. Eventually, he had to leave school again and be tutored at home. Keith's insurance would not pay for a second IV Ig treatment. The family was fortunate to find an "angel" donor who stepped in to cover the cost.

Keith's mom was devastated when, in spite of a second order from the neurologist, her local hospital refused to repeat IV Ig. The doctors did not feel the treatment was appropriate for his condition. She contacted me, and I explained that you cannot force a doctor or hospital to render any particular type of treatment. I suggested that she consider treatment at an infusion center instead. Coram is a well-known chain of infusion centers located throughout the country with a site in Falmouth, Maine. She contacted Coram and confirmed that

IV Ig is very expensive and not always covered by insurance, so be sure to check with your insurance company before agreeing to the procedure.

it would follow through on an IV Ig treatment prescribed by an out-of-state physician. Whether an order or prescription from an out-of-state physician can be honored in a different state is a matter of state regulation. For example, a Florida physician has to sign off on medical orders for treatment in Florida. Other states will permit an out-of-state physician's order to be followed.

On the morning of the procedure, Keith rested comfortably in a chair that resembled a Lay-Z-Boy recliner. The nurse patiently sought the best vein in his arm. Once the vein was located and the needle inserted, the procedure began. The IV Ig solution is thick, and the body will draw fluids from the body to help process it through the liver, so a patient who has not had sufficient liquids can end up dehydrated. For that reason, Keith's doctor had ordered an infusion of saline solution to begin thirty minutes prior to starting the IV Ig. If the doctor does not order the saline infusion, then the patient must be sure to drink plenty of liquids. Some patients have problems with nausea and headaches following the IV Ig infusion, so to help prevent those symptoms, the doctor had also ordered ibuprofen, benadryl, and Zofran fifteen minutes prior to the infusion of the IV Ig. Ibuprofen helps reduce inflammation so it may help tighten the BBB. Benadryl helps avert any allergic reaction the child may have to the new proteins contained in the infusion. Zofran helps with nausea. Once the IV Ig infusion started, Keith's blood pressure, weight, and temperature were checked every fifteen minutes for the first hour, then every thirty minutes for the next two hours, and then once an hour until completion. It was a long, two-day process, lasting six hours each day, with an additional hour at the end for a final infusion of saline.

Keith was relaxed and talkative during his infusion and pleased to share his story for this book. He was hopeful that he would respond well to the IV Ig, which he described as "one poke to being perfect." He said he needed help with his aggression and his hand washing. I asked him if there were any thoughts he'd like me to pass along to other children who might be waiting for IV Ig and somewhat concerned. He said, "The IV fluid is thick like syrup so drink plenty of water to keep headaches away, the nurses are nice and there to help. Movies, games, puzzles, and naps help pass the time. I was able to have my meals at their regular times, and my nurse even had a snack basket for me when I needed one."

Keith's nurse showed me the acute infusion reaction box she had full of medications just in case a patient might have a severe allergic reaction to the IV Ig. Those reactions are extremely rare, and she had not yet experienced one with a patient. Keith's mother carried an EpiPen with her. An EpiPen is used to treat life threatening allergic reactions and the doctor had ordered it as a safety measure. It's a shot of epinephrine injected directly into the patient's muscle. In a severe reaction the patient can't breathe because his airways close, and the shot will open the airways pending arrival of an ambulance. If you are prescribed an EpiPen, you need to make sure you know how to use it. The written instructions in the box are not clear, but your physician can guide you. There are also numerous instructional videos posted on YouTube.

While Keith was infused, we talked about all the things I had learned while researching this book and what other changes that I thought might help Keith's body to fight the disorder. We reviewed many of the suggestions contained in chapter 6, "Nutritional Considerations." While Keith's mom took notes, Keith periodically nodded with, "We're going to do that," or, "That makes sense."

Keith's mom mentioned that they are considering a tonsillectomy for Keith.

Keith's mom got back in touch with me about a month later. He had a good initial response to the IV Ig, but it did not last. She was sad to report that his behaviors had returned.

SUMMING IT UP

PANDAS requires a multi-treatment approach. One doctor may be able to provide some of what's needed, but it's doubtful that any one doctor is going to be able to do it all. To attack the infection, reduce inflammation while building the immune system, and manage the psychiatric symptoms you will need treatment providers capable of prescribing medication. Helping your child with the skills she needs to manage her behavioral symptoms while she heals will probably require engaging a psychologist. Section III of this book helps you in assembling your child's treatment team, choosing the members, and working effectively with them. But first let's cover the behavioral and nutritional interventions that may help.

BIG IDEAS FROM CHAPTER FOUR

❑ The four aspects to treating PANDAS are:
  attacking the infection
  reducing inflammation and building the immune system
  addressing the psychiatric symptoms
  developing behavioral skills.
❑ Infections are addressed through antibiotics, blood procedures, and sometimes tonsillectomies.
❑ Reducing inflammation may be helped through over-the-counter anti-inflammatories or by prescription medications.
❑ Building the immune system can be helped with dietary changes.
❑ Psychiatric symptoms are treated through psychotropic medications. *(continued)*

❑ Behavioral skills are built with cognitive behavioral therapy.
❑ A child with PANDAS will most likely need multiple treatment providers to address all these goals.

Cognitive Behavioral Therapy

5

Dear Beth,
My son was sick for almost a year before we found out what was wrong. He was getting so much better for so many months, but now it seems the medicine has stopped working. When he starts a behavior we try to have him stop and gain control over it. We aren't disciplining because of the behavior, but we will tell him to stop doing it, and we have a few different things we have him do to try to help him regain control. Do you have any ideas for us? Do you think we need to change the antibiotic?
Stuck

Dear Stuck,
Have you tried cognitive behavioral therapy (CBT)? He may need professional help to master his behaviors. I honestly do not think these are skills you can offer him without input and direction from a therapist who is trained to offer CBT. Many children improve, but then hit a behavioral plateau. Often, what they need is CBT.
Beth

Overcoming Problem Behaviors

Children with PANDAS are plagued by rituals and behaviors, which can be mild or disabling depending upon the severity and duration of the illness. When PANDAS is recognized early, and the behaviors are mild, it's possible that they will fade with appropriate medication. For most children, although the behaviors may improve, they do not usually just "go away." The children will need to work hard to

FACT:
Cognitive behavioral therapy is not talk therapy. CBT consists of a specific set of assigned tasks that—when practiced consistently—are designed to enable the patient to overcome his troubling behaviors.

conquer the behaviors and patterns that have become an integrated part of them and their everyday lives. The type of therapy specifically designed to address the problem is called cognitive behavioral therapy: CBT.

I use fingernail biting as an analogy because I bit mine when I was a kid. Even when I desperately wanted to stop biting my nails, it was incredibly hard to stop. My mom put bad-tasting stuff on my nails, but I got used to it. I tried wearing Band-Aids on the tips of my fingers, but those "fell off." I had to work hard to consciously make myself stop putting my hand to my mouth. And even when I had "stopped biting" I still suffered the consequences. My nails were weak and splitting for years. It was a long time before those last remnants of nail biting were over. I think that's a minor version of what your children experience. The troublesome behaviors have developed into nasty habits, and it's going to be hard work to break them. Even when the behaviors have been substantially eliminated, the remnants may stick around for a while. Often times, your child will need the help of a therapist specially trained in CBT.

This chapter explains CBT and describes an excellent program so that you will have the information you will need when you begin to seek CBT treatment for your child.

What Is CBT?

FACT:
"Evidence-based practice" means that the best available evidence gained from the scientific method is applied to clinical practice.

CBT is a systematic approach to tackling dysfunctional behaviors through methods proven to change them. It's an evidence-based practice that can cover many areas of emotional and behavioral problems, but for PANDAS children the focus of CBT is its application to ritualized, obsessive-compulsive behaviors. Many patients with OCD recognize that their obsessions and compulsions are irrational. With the help of a good therapist, CBT will help them stop repeating the rituals and conquer the behaviors.

The CBT therapeutic approach is the same for all children suffering with OCD. It does not matter whether an infection triggered the disorder or if the child was simply born with the condition. It only matters that the behaviors are so much a part of your child that they negatively impact everyday life. OCD is a giant burden to carry. You want your child to get rid of that burden as quickly as possible and CBT can help.

The keys to making CBT work are prolonged, repetitive, and graduated exposures coupled with preventing the rituals that follow the exposures.

Timing. Consistent with most things in life, timing matters. Part of the solution is introducing CBT at the right time. If you introduce CBT before your child is capable of engaging in the therapy, it will be a waste of time and resources and may cause her to feel like a failure. The analogy I use is that you can't correct a child's penmanship if she can't hold a pen. By the same token, you want to put CBT in place while recovery is on the upswing. Otherwise, the child may get discouraged about whether she'll ever get better and may lose incentive. There's a delicate balance between pressure and challenge, but you will know when it's the right time for your child. I can't offer a timetable for starting CBT because each child is different. I can tell you it took Sammy about three and a half months on the correct treatment with antibiotics before he was able to engage meaningfully in CBT. He was also well enough by then to be personally determined to fully recover. Start exploring your options for CBT even before your child is ready to participate because it may take some effort to locate the right person and program. If you have it lined up in advance, you'll be all set to go just as soon as your child is ready.

Advice from an Expert: Bradley C. Reimann, PhD. To assist me in understanding CBT, I met with Bradley C. Reimann, PhD. He is the director of the OCD Center and Cognitive Behavioral Therapy Services at Rogers Memorial Hospital in Oconomowoc, Wisconsin. Rogers is a private psychiatric hospital that offers nationally recognized residential and intensive outpatient programs (IOP) for adults and children afflicted with a range of disorders including OCD, anxiety, eating disorders, conversion disorders, and addiction. Rogers Hospital offers the only residential program in the country for children with OCD who are under sixteen years old. Dr. Reimann began working with children who have OCD in 1987, and he has been with Rogers since 1997. He estimates that his largely successful programs have treated over one thousand children with OCD over the past twenty-five years. In short, this is a guy who knows what he's talking about. By reading what Dr. Reimann has to say about CBT, you will be in a better position to evaluate the therapist and program you are considering for your child.

Although patients at Rogers Hospital are treated with a combination of medication and therapy, this chapter will concentrate only on the therapeutic aspect because medication treatments were covered in chapter 4, "Medical Treatment."

Developing hierarchies. Dr. Reimann's first step is to develop hierarchies of what causes the child anxiety on a scale of zero to seven. Zero are the behaviors that cause no anxiety whatsoever. Seven is the most anxiety-producing behavior the patient could ever possibly imagine. For example, touching the knob that flushes the toilet at home might be a four, while touching one in a public restroom might be a seven. Within the hierarchies, Dr. Reimann gets very specific about finding out the details of what causes the trouble. He may learn that one child's contamination fear is germs, but for another the fear is radiation. Another child may be okay with doorknobs inside the home, but not outside. Specific exercises or exposures are then generated for each level of hierarchies and tailored to the particular fear.

> **FACT:**
> *A hierarchy ranks each cause of anxiety on a scale of zero to seven.*

Patients begin their program at Rogers Hospital with "the threes." Ones, twos, and threes are considered challenging but manageable anxieties, things that patients should be able to push themselves to do. Fours and fives are iffy. Some patients may be able to push themselves to do a four or five, others will not. Sixes and sevens are impossible. The complexity and severity of the OCD will determine the extent of the hierarchies and the level of care that your child requires.

Exposure and ritual prevention. Based on the hierarchies, Dr. Reimann develops a set of two-part exercises for the patient: exposure and ritual prevention (ERP). The hierarchies dictate how the two parts will be implemented. The basic program is that patients will be exposed to the thing that produces anxiety, and the rituals that the exposure prompts will be avoided. As the child works her way up the ladder from threes to fours and eventually conquering fives, those things that were a seven keep dropping down.

> **FACT:**
> *There are two parts to CBT: exposure and ritual prevention ("ERP").*

If a child is afraid of touching doorknobs (six) but less afraid of holding a pen (three), the exposure might begin with pens. She will repeatedly practice holding a pen, not washing her hands before or after holding the pen, and not washing the pen itself. Once she has mastered pens, she will move on to an item from level four. Keep in mind, the item on level four has now dropped down to a three. Eventually, the patient will work her way up to tackling doorknobs. The program for doorknobs is the same as it was for the earlier items. She doesn't just touch a doorknob, she stands there and holds it for a while. Then she does it repeatedly, and she does not wash the knob or wash her hand before or after touching the knob.

Dr. Reimann is careful to make sure the process is not overwhelming. He titrates the exposures so that the exercises are challenging but manageable. Dr. Reimann feels that approaching exposures in a graduated fashion helps; less patients drop out or refuse to participate in the therapy. He compares it with training for a marathon where the runner slowly builds to run the distance.

Dr. Reimann pointed out that during recovery there will be selective avoidance. If the patient's dad knows that doorknobs are a problem, then the dad will hold the door until his child is ready to do it alone. The only glitch is "sometimes life throws you a six," said Dr. Reimann. For those instances, he encourages the patient to try reducing the ritual. If confronted with a doorknob before the patient is ready, he might suggest a two- or three-minute hand washing instead of the usual ten-minute ritual.

> **FACT:**
> *ERP exercises should be challenging, but manageable. Too much, too soon may be overwhelming.*

What the doctor says:

"I want my patients to confront the things that scare them, but in a way that encourages success."

Bradley C. Reimann, PhD
Rogers Memorial Hospital
Oconomowoc, WI

Dr. Reimann tries to assign a manageable number of exposures as "homework" so that the exposures can be repeated at least five times each day. During the exposure, the goal is to have the child's anxiety drop by at least half. When the child holds a doorknob that's dropped down to a four, it might take five minutes before the doorknob becomes a two, but she will get there and then the exposure can end. During the exposure, the clinician tracks the level of anxiety but does not give "you're okay" reassurance. According to Dr. Reimann, reassurance fuels the problem. The child needs to learn for herself that she will be okay. Encouragement is offered: "You're doing great, hang in there, this might be a big step, but I know you can do this, your anxiety is coming down." After the child does this five times in one day, chances are her anxiety level at approaching the unwashed doorknob will no longer be a four. The goal is to establish zeros as quickly as possible. Dr. Reimann's goal is to get the child through 70 percent of her individual hierarchy and then discharge her to a lower level of care.

FACT: *Reassurance fuels the problem; what you want to offer instead is encouragement.*

Rogers Memorial Hospital has found that 83 percent of patients who achieve 70 percent of their hierarchy will then either maintain their gains or continue to get better.

Common obsessions and compulsions. According to Dr. Reimann, there are broad categories of behaviors that generally trouble OCD patients. Examples of common obsessions are contamination, doubting, religious, harming, exactness, symmetry, and sexual. The obsessions lead to the common compulsions, which include washing, cleaning, checking, counting, praying, reassurance seeking, ordering, and arranging. Where the behavior fits into an individual's hierarchy is different for each patient. For example, because contamination and washing are common problems, doorknobs often pose difficulty. For one patient, touching a doorknob may be a two, but it might be a five for someone else. Within the category of contamination and washing, there will also be issues with touching light switches, faucets, and public toilets, and hugs or shaking people's hands. For children who doubt and check, this will include, "Did I finish that math problem, did I lock my locker, did I zip my book bag?" Dr. Reimann points out that harming obsessions (constantly worrying about hurting another person or an animal) are one of the most misunderstood areas of OCD; a child consumed with harming obsessions is one of the last people in the world who will ever harm anyone.

Outpatient treatment. Dr. Reimann believes that the vast majority of OCD patients do not need residential treatment. It's a very treatable condition and most of it can be done in an outpatient or intensive outpatient (IOP) setting provided that the quality of the program is up to par and the quantity is sufficient. For children, the level of the disability and thus appropriate care is determined by looking at how the child is functioning at home, school, and with friends. Functioning can range from a child who has some difficulty at school, to a child hanging on by a thread, or one who has not been in school for six months. The complexity of the OCD may range from fairly circumscribed—just a few obsessions—to those who have them all. There may also be other disorders involved that add to the complexity, including anxiety disorders, an eating disorder, and depression. All of these considerations will lead to a determination of what level of treatment your child needs. Quality and quantity are crucial to treatment.

An effective ERP program. According to Dr. Reimann, "dabbling" will not be effective for OCD, and a good program should move quickly.

What the doctor says:

"It's ERP 24/7 from a therapy standpoint. Talking about the anxieties is not productive, and doing exposures here and there will be ineffective."

Bradley C. Reimann, PhD

Within the first hour of an outpatient session, the therapist should be able to gather enough information to confirm the diagnosis and generally outline a plan for treatment. Optimally, both parents and the child should attend the first session. During that first family session, it will not be possible to develop the individual hierarchies, but you should have a good idea of what the therapist's overall plan will be. By the second session, the therapist should be developing hierarchies. Developing the hierarchies at Rogers Memorial takes roughly three hours and by the fourth hour exposures are being assigned. "Everyone needs to know what's involved, and at least one parent must be involved at every step of the process," said Dr. Reimann. "Out of necessity, the parents must become a bit of armchair behavioral therapists themselves because most of the work has to be done at home." The parents must develop the skills needed to make sure their child gets the "ERP homework" done. Parents need to know the basics, and the outcomes are so much better when they are involved.

Choosing a Therapist. Taking the child with you to multiple appointments while you screen therapists is not the best approach. Do some preliminary screening by telephone, and take your child along only when you think you may have found the final candidate. If the therapist is not willing to spend fifteen minutes on the telephone talking with you and answering your questions for free, look elsewhere. Obviously there will be some variation, but if the therapist you are considering cannot outline a program with specificity or the outline is for a program that will move substantially slower than outlined above, you need to find someone else. You are looking for someone who can quickly implement the exposures and ritual preventions that will point your child in the right direction. Take your time and be thorough about screening. You are selecting a person who will become a pivotal person in your child's life so you want to be reasonably certain that you've made the right choice. Dr. Reimann pointed out, "Many people take more time to pick a contractor than they do to pick a clinician."

The person you're interviewing to work with your child should be talking about hierarchies, exposure and ritual prevention (ERP), and the Yale-Brown Obsessive-Compulsive Scale (Y-BOCS or CY-BOCS). Some capable therapists do still use the older term of exposure and response prevention rather than ritual prevention. If the rest of the information is what you want to hear, then don't let the use of that term be the decisive factor.

For help finding a good therapist, visit the "Treatment Provider" page on the website for the International OCD Foundation (ocfoundation.org). Start by looking for someone who is a Behavioral Therapy Training Institute (BTTI) graduate or faculty member. The page also has some good tips about questions to ask a therapist when you are screening to find the right person. Among other things, you will want to know:

- ❑ How quickly will the hierarchies be developed?
- ❑ How soon will the child be assigned exposures?
- ❑ How many people has your candidate treated with OCD?
- ❑ What are your candidate's outcomes?

There are also a couple of outpatient clinics associated with hospitals that you might want to explore. One is at Massachusetts General Hospital, and another is at UCLA.

 What the doctor says:

"If parents try to handle this themselves, start with the most tolerable anxieties and try building from there; but I do advise to find a good therapist."

Bradley C. Reimann, PhD

SUMMING IT UP

From reading this chapter, you now understand CBT, why it works, and what constitutes an effective CBT program. You know the qualities you need to find in a therapist and are ready to do the appropriate screening. Most children do not need inpatient treatment, but for those who do it is invaluable. If your child is well enough to be able to make progress with outpatient therapy, but you cannot find someone qualified, perhaps you should consider the intensive outpatient program at Rogers Hospital. Traveling to Wisconsin and spending a month in a hotel may not sound ideal, but compared to spending nonproductive months seeking ineffective treatment, it may well be worth considering.

BIG IDEAS FROM CHAPTER FIVE

- ❏ Cognitive Behavioral Therapy (CBT) is an evidence-based practice comprised of targeted behavioral exercises.
- ❏ The goal of the exercises is to enable patients with OCD to overcome their behaviors.
- ❏ There are two parts to CBT exercises: exposures and ritual preventions (ERP).
- ❏ A hierarchy is a ranking of the anxieties that plague the child and trigger the OCD behaviors.
- ❏ Your child's hierarchies will dictate the ERP exercises that will be assigned.
- ❏ A good therapist will assign exercises that are challenging, but not overwhelming.
- ❏ Children should be encouraged, but not reassured, when engaging in ERP.
- ❏ CBT is hard work; it should be introduced when your child is well enough to engage meaningfully in the treatment.
- ❏ A successful CBT program will start with less challenging anxieties and move steadily to the more difficult areas.
- ❏ Talking about anxieties will not overcome OCD behaviors.

Nutritional Considerations

6

Dear Beth,
I've noticed that when my daughter is at her worst, she wants bread, especially white bread, and lots of it. My instinct tells me there's a problem with the bread, and I've read that we sometimes crave foods that aren't good for us. Could I be right about the bread and PANDAS?
Intuitive Mom

Dear Intuitive,
White bread quickly breaks down into sugar. Sugar feeds bacteria and causes inflammation. As the bacteria grows stronger, the immune system will produce more antibodies to fight the infection, and the increased inflammation will enable those antibodies to easily cross into the brain. So, yes, you're exactly right; white bread is probably tied to the behavioral exacerbations.
Beth

What Your Child Eats Is Important

Paying attention to your child's nutrition is just as important as understanding the disorder, securing medical treatment, compiling records, and working with doctors, because appropriate nutrition will help manage the disorder.

There are three goals when it comes to feeding your PANDAS child:

- ❏ starve the bacteria
- ❏ reduce inflammation
- ❏ boost the immune system

71

Ideally, all the foods your child eats should further one of those goals, and your child should not eat anything that may have the opposite effect.

This chapter will explain how diet impacts the health of your child. It will help you make knowledgeable decisions about which foods your child should eat, and which foods your child should avoid. One of the best things about nutritional intervention is that you don't need to wait for a doctor to write a prescription. These are all steps that you can take right away simply by visiting the grocery store.

Digestion and Nourishment

Because you want your child's digestive system to work as hard for your child as you are working, understanding the basics of that system is a necessary first step. Here's a primer.

The *digestive tract* consists of the mouth, throat (esophagus), stomach, small intestine, large intestine (also called the colon), rectum, and anus. When you think of the digestive tract, picture your food moving through the body. First it goes in through the mouth and then down the throat to the stomach. Once food passes through the stomach, it arrives in the small intestine, where nutrients are absorbed into the body. The balance, fiber and waste, passes through the large intestines (or colon) and then out of the body through the rectum or anus.

FACT:

The vast majority of the immune system resides in the intestinal tract. If the intestinal tract is not healthy, the immune system will not function properly.

The stomach, together with both intestines, is called the gastrointestinal or GI tract. The small and large intestines, without the stomach, are called the *intestinal tract*. The vast majority of the immune system (as much as 60 to 80 percent) resides in the intestinal tract, so maintaining a healthy intestinal tract, or *"gut,"* is essential to having a healthy immune system. PANDAS children have immune systems that are not functioning as well as those of other children. By helping to make sure your child's intestinal tract is healthy, you will be helping your child battle back PANDAS.

When your child first eats her food, it is not in a form that can nourish the body. It must be continually broken down into smaller pieces and eventually molecules so that they can be absorbed into the blood and carried to cells throughout the body. *Digestion* is the process of turning food into molecules that can be used to nourish cells and provide energy. It begins when food is chewed and swallowed. As food moves through the system it is continually changed into smaller components by layers of smooth muscles that line the digestive tract and by digestive juices produced by the liver and pancreas. When food reaches the small intestine, nutrients are absorbed by the villi that send them into the

FACT:
Villi are tiny, fingerlike projections that line the wall of the small intestine, absorb nutrients, and send them into the body.

body. *Villi* are tiny, fingerlike projections that protrude from the lining of the intestinal wall. When I think of villi, I picture seaweed waving from the ocean floor. If your child's body is not able to turn her food into nutrients, or if she is not eating foods that supply the nutrients that the villi need to absorb, then her intestinal tract will not be functioning properly.

1. Starve the Bacteria. The first thing you want to do for a PANDAS child is starve the bacteria. All bacteria thrive on sugar. Sugar is the main source of energy for the body, but blood sugar levels have to remain appropriate. Most people are generally familiar with this in the context of diabetes, but it's important for infections, too. Every time your child eats something sugary, she causes her blood sugar to rise, thus offering a food source for the bacteria that is causing her infection. And as the bacteria grow and become more powerful, they will demand more sugar, resulting in a craving. Simply put, the more sugar your child eats, the more sugar she is going to want. So you need to take immediate steps to eliminate as much sugar as possible.

FACT:
Your child's bacterial infection thrives on sugar.

Sugars are also called *simple carbohydrates*. Ice cream, cookies, cake, candies, candy bars, soda, syrup, sugary cereals, and junk food are all simple carbohydrates. Sometimes I hear parents say they are reluctant to eliminate these because "it's all she'll eat." Now you know why: because the bacteria are calling the shots. You need to break that cycle. A recovering alcoholic cannot have alcohol in the house. For a PANDAS patient, it is the sugar that needs to go.

Simple carbohydrates also include fruits, but fruits also have vitamins, fiber, and important nutrients. So when your child craves something sweet, give her fruit. Fruit juice is a healthier alternative than soda, but keep in mind that a cup of apple juice has six times the sugar of the apple itself. Therefore, if your child will eat the whole apple instead of drinking a cup of apple juice, that will be the best.

You not only have to eliminate the obvious sugars, such as cake and candy, but you also need to eliminate foods that the body quickly and easily breaks down into sugar. When foods quickly break down into sugar, it creates a spike in blood sugar, making it a friendly place for bacteria to thrive. As a rule of thumb, the foods that quickly break down into sugar are the "white foods," so avoid them as much as possible. For example, there is nothing nutritional about white bread. It immediately breaks down into sugar and the more white bread she eats the more sugar she will want. If your child must have white bread, try having her eat it with nuts or another food that will slow down the digestive process and help avoid the spike in sugar. White potatoes and white rice also quickly break down into sugar. Try substituting sweet potatoes and brown rice. If transitioning from white rice to brown is a problem, begin by mixing half and half. Jasmine brown rice is similar in consistency to white rice and might be a good place to start. If you don't have fifty minutes to devote to cooking a pot of brown rice, the ten-minute versions are excellent alternatives.

FACT:

By weaning your child off sugar, and the "white foods" that break down into sugar, you will be making it harder for the infection to survive.

The reason diabetics often have a hard time with infections is because their blood is high in sugar. You want to create the opposite environment: a body system that is not a friendly place for infections to thrive. Your child may not be eating much at all, and it may not be possible to clear out all the sugar overnight, but by staying persistent you can successfully wean most of it from your child's diet. Sugar not only feeds the bacteria, but also has been linked to suppressing the immune system by interfering with the body's ability to attack bacteria. There is no upside to sugar. As you'll read below, it contributes to inflammation and high sugar diets can contribute to a yeast overgrowth that may lead to "leaky gut syndrome." The more you can eliminate sugar from your child's diet, the healthier she will become.

2. Reduce Inflammation. PANDAS is an autoimmune disorder and inflammation is part of the problem. Not only does inflammation make the blood-brain barrier more permeable, but it also inhibits the absorption of nutrients. Inflammation can be reduced through a two-prong method: eating an anti-inflammatory diet and avoiding foods that may cause an allergic reaction.

FACT: Inflammation makes the blood-brain barrier more permeable and inhibits the absorption of nutrients.

An anti-inflammatory diet. You want your child to eat the foods that fight inflammation, and have him stay away from those that increase inflammation.

If you Google "top ten anti-inflammatory foods," you will find:

- kelp (which you can get in granulized form and sprinkle on soups)
- turmeric
- ginger and garlic
- wild salmon
- shiitake mushroom
- green tea
- papaya and pineapple
- berries (blueberries, cranberries, goji berries, strawberries, and raspberries)
- extra virgin olive oil
- broccoli, sweet potato, and spinach

Grocery shopping from a list of anti-inflammatory foods and then including them in your child's diet will help your child in his recovery, and don't forget to pick up a bottle of fish oil capsules.

What the doctor says:

"By looking on the label, you will be able to see the amount of Omega 3 per capsule of fish oil and figure out how many capsules are needed to reach 2000 to 3000 milligrams per day."

Robert Sears, MD, FAAP (Dr. Bob)

Equally important is to stop bringing home the inflammatory foods. If you Google "top ten inflammatory foods," you will find sugar at the top of the list. Also on that list will be:

- ❑ dairy (milk, cheese, yogurt)
- ❑ common cooking oils (use olive oil instead)
- ❑ deep fried foods, feedlot fed meat (beef, pork and chicken)
- ❑ red and processed meat (such as sausage and salami)
- ❑ alcohol
- ❑ refined grains (white rice, white flour, white bread)
- ❑ food additives such as monosodium glutamate and aspartame
- ❑ gluten
- ❑ nuts, eggs, and nightshade vegetables (such as tomatoes and potatoes).

Avoiding allergic reactions. Doing everything you can to eliminate the possibility of an allergic reaction is a good step, too, because allergic reactions are, by nature, inflammatory. It's easy to picture inflammation when it happens on the skin, just think of poison ivy. Most of us know that for some people bee stings and peanuts can cause such a severe reaction in the immune system that it can be life threatening; it's called *anaphylactic shock*. It's easy to identify an allergic reaction when the skin is broken out in hives or if a person is choking and gasping for breath; then we do our best to avoid the *allergen* (the thing causing the reaction). An allergic child doesn't play in a poison ivy patch, any more than a person with a peanut allergy tries eating a few to see if it happens again. But when inflammation happens wholly inside the body, we can't see it. So allergic reactions to food can be entirely overlooked.

Two well-known *dietary allergens* are *gluten* and *casein*:

❑ Gluten is found in all products containing wheat, barley, rye, and sometimes oats.
❑ Casein is found in all dairy products such as milk, butter, and cheese.

Gluten and casein may be causing inflammation of which you are not aware, so it's worth exploring gluten- and casein-free diets.

Gluten has become more of a problem as wheat and similar grains have been genetically engineered to be hardier and more resistant to bugs and mold. Coupled with pesticides sprayed on the grains, our bodies sometimes have a tough time managing. Moreover, the symptoms of a gluten allergy may not be recognized and go undetected for years. If your child is allergic to gluten, his immune system will produce antibodies that cross-react with the tissue of the small intestine, and one result will be inflammation. A more unfortunate result may be *celiac disease*. Celiac disease is potentially fatal when it destroys the villi that line the small intestine, thus preventing the body from absorbing nutrients. Even if your child is only sensitive to the gluten, without a full allergic reaction, the immune system will be at work producing antibodies.

Eliminating gluten may accomplish two things:

❑ the immune system can rest from fighting gluten
❑ the inflammation that may be the byproduct of that battle will no longer be present

With the immune system no longer diverted by fighting the gluten, it may be better able to fight your child's infection. And reducing inflammation will help to seal the BBB. For these reasons, PANDAS

 What the doctor says:

"I treat the whole child, and I find that many are gluten intolerant. It is well known that gluten intolerance can trigger autoimmune disease, and that's what PANDAS is."

Ali Carine, DO

patients often benefit from a gluten-free diet. Moreover, there is no downside to eliminating gluten; the body does not need it.

The symptoms of gluten intolerance can be as simple as a stomachache. When my friend Justine Tanguay's five-year-old complained of bellyaches on and off for a couple of months, she suspected that he was allergic to something he was eating. She had the pediatrician run a full series of blood tests for food allergies. The child turned out to be gluten intolerant. With a gluten-free diet in place, his bellyaches are gone. "I think parents really need to pay attention when their kids say they have bellyaches," she said, "and if the parents can't afford the tests, I'd try eliminating gluten and casein to see what happens." As you will learn when you read the full interviews with Dr. Carine and Dr. Sears in the appendix, they both recommend trying a gluten-free diet even without blood work. Much like treating suspected cases of PANDAS with antibiotics, the question is not so much what the blood work says, but whether your child responds.

Casein is another common dietary allergen. Casein is a protein that is contained in the milk of humans, cows, goats, and sheep, but structurally it is different in each mammal. Cow milk is what presents the problem, and 80 percent of the proteins in cow milk are casein. The different structure of the protein in various mammals may explain why people who are allergic to cow milk can often tolerate goat milk as a substitute.

FACT:
Gluten and casein are common food allergens that are often overlooked.

When the immune system produces antibodies to casein, it can trigger inflammation, stomach problems, skin rashes, hives, and even breathing difficulties. Reactions to casein can be slight or severe. If severe, it can be as dangerous as a peanut allergy, and the patient may have to carry a shot of epinephrine in case he suffers anaphylactic shock. Even slicing meat with a knife that has been used to slice cheese may cause a reaction in a highly allergic person. If the allergy is less severe, the symptoms may not be noticed or they may be excused to a tummy ache or other causes. In either case, if your child is allergic to casein, his production of antibodies will cause inflammation. Some researchers believe that as much as 60 percent of the world's population can't digest cow milk so it's worth considering whether it might be contributing to inflammation in your child's system.

By eliminating casein (as with gluten), you will be giving the immune system an opportunity to rest and inflammation will decrease. Lactose-free milk will not solve the problem, because that only eliminates the sugar found in milk. Goat, soy, rice, and almond milk are all alternatives to cow milk so you might want to experiment until you find one your child likes. They will not taste the same as cow milk. They will taste different, but different can be good. Most of these alternative milks are readily available at grocery stores and even Wal-mart carries a good selection.

Given that fact that the immune system of a PANDAS child is already struggling, reducing gluten and casein—even if you do not manage to eliminate them—makes good common sense.

3. Boost the Immune System. The immune system is what defends us against the millions of bacteria, viruses, microbes, toxins, and parasites that constantly try to invade our bodies. We need that system strong and ready to fight. The intestinal tract, or "gut," is home to the vast majority of the immune system, so you want that home to be a place where the immune system can flourish. You do everything you can to make sure your personal home is a place where your children will flourish. You need to make that same effort toward your child's intestinal tract. Making sure that your child's digestive system is well supported is not only important to recovering from PANDAS, but to keeping your child healthy when he recovers. Once you get rid of PANDAS, the immune system can be your greatest ally in making sure it never comes back. Let's talk about how to make sure it's always ready to work on your child's behalf.

Probiotic bacteria and digestive enzymes. Humans need good bacteria and digestive enzymes in their gut to help turn otherwise indigestible foods into a form that is digestible. Without these good bacteria (*probiotics*) and proteins (*enzymes*), your digestive system cannot process food into nutrients. One of the concerns about antibiotics is that they may wipe out the good bacteria along with the bad. If that happens, then the intestinal tract is out of balance and, for example, yeast can become a problem.

We all have yeast in our bodies. It normally resides in the

FACT:

A "leaky gut" is when yeast penetrates the intestinal wall, allowing particles to escape directly into the body. Yeast overgrowths can be caused by high sugar diets and when antibiotics wipe out the good bacteria in the gut.

intestinal tract. Levels of yeast are kept in check by the immune system and probiotics. If antibiotics kill off the probiotics and the immune system becomes weakened, then yeast may grow unchecked. High sugar diets also contribute to an overgrowth of yeast. When the yeast is not properly checked, the overgrown yeast may penetrate the intestinal wall, causing it and other particles to escape and be absorbed into the body. This is called a "leaky gut." So particularly while your child is on antibiotics, make sure you are replacing the good bacteria that may be inadvertently wiped out by antibiotics. You want to be certain that what belongs in the gut, stays there.

One way to help support the digestive system is through probiotic supplements and dietary enzymes. Another way is to feed your child foods that are rich in the things she needs. One such food is miso soup. If you enjoy cooking, you can of course make your own miso paste and then the soup. Alternatively, you can go to the refrigerator section of the health food store and find the paste to make miso soup. By mixing the paste with hot water, you can offer your child a tasty miso soup that is loaded with probiotics and digestive enzymes.

Fermented foods are another excellent way to provide probiotic support. They will help feed the probiotics already in your system. Sauerkraut and sour pickles that you can buy at the health food

What the doctor says:

"The child should take probiotics when on antibiotics, but read the label carefully. Some contain strep species. For PANDAS, I think it's best to steer clear of any kind of strep at all. If the child develops a yeast overgrowth, I prescribe Nystatin. It can safely be taken for many months without worry about side effects."

Robert Sears, MD, FAAP (Dr. Bob)

store will do the trick. If you are adventurous in the kitchen, you might want to ferment your own cabbage and root vegetables (such as carrots, onion, and radishes) with sea salt by following a kimchi recipe.

Yogurt is also a good source of probiotics, but for reasons explained in the section above, you might prefer for your child to have non-dairy yogurt such as that made with soy or another substitute for cow milk.

Supplying Nutrients. You want your child to eat *nutrient-dense foods*. Nutrient-dense foods have a high level of nutrients compared to the number of calories they contain. These nutrients include vitamins, essential fatty acids, fiber, and minerals. If you Google "nutrient dense foods" you can find lists, but generally your child needs as many whole foods as possible: fresh fruits and vegetables, raw nuts, very little processed food (meaning food that comes in a package).

You may want to consider using a juicer and blender, particularly if your children are difficult with fruits and vegetables. Kids think it's fun to drop fruits and veggies into juicers and blenders, so they'll want to help while you supervise. Juices are a terrific way to easily deliver nutrients. Your child can certainly eat five carrots. But creating a five carrot juice containing other vegetables and a piece of fruit will be the fastest way to deliver a much needed boost to the immune system.

Buy a juicer. Delivering vegetables in liquid form is one of the easiest and fastest ways that you can deliver nutrient-dense foods to your child.

Carrots are a good base for juices, then add any combination of other vegetables: cucumber, kale, celery, parsley, avocado, peppers, and chard are possibilities. If your juicer won't extract juices from the leafy greens, wrap them tightly around each other before dropping them in the juicer. Drop in pineapple, apple, or pear to sweeten it up, and if you include a bit of fresh ginger, you will have introduced a natural anti-inflammatory. It's best to buy organic when you intend to eat the skins of the fruits and vegetables. If that isn't possible, wash them well or take the skins off before dropping them into the juicer.

Smoothies are easy to make in a blender. Some health food stores have specialty items like dates rolled in coconut that add a great taste. Soy yogurt with bananas and anti-inflammatory berries is a scrumptious way to help your child. There are many brands of delicious brands of soy yogurt available including Stonyfield and Trader Joe's.

Nutritional Advice from an Expert

I asked my friend Meg Wolff how she would feed a PANDAS child because she is a national advocate for the relationship between health and diet. When Meg lost a leg and a breast to cancer, she took a careful look at the relationship between her disease and what she ate. It caused her to completely change her eating habits. She reversed her condition and now, twelve years later, she remains cancer free. She firmly believes that by eating a healthy diet, she healed her immune system and helped stave off cancer. When I asked Meg about PANDAS, she was ready with an answer because her daughter had recurrent bouts with strep as a ten-year-old. "I'd starve the bacteria, first," she said, "by eliminating sugar; then I'd concentrate on feeding nutrient-rich food and eliminating animal protein." By animal protein, Meg is referring to beef, chicken, fish, cheese, and eggs.

For breakfast, she fed her daughter oatmeal and a cup of miso soup. But if your child insists on cereal, Meg suggests a brand called Erewhon. For pancakes, she recommends mixes from Bob's Red Mill. If your child wants syrup, which ideally would be best to eliminate entirely due to sugar, she recommends brown rice syrup or real maple syrup instead of artificial syrups. She suggests reducing beef, chicken, fish, cheese, and eggs (animal proteins) by at least one-third. In their place, she'd add grains such as millet, quinoa, and brown rice as well as beans and soy products, for example tofu.

"If you learn five new recipes for entrees that become your 'go-to' recipes, it's a great way to get started," said Meg. "If you are going gluten or wheat free, you just need to be sure to use a rice product instead of wheat," she added. "And remember to use wheat-free tamari for your soy sauce."

Five of the simplest recipes from her book *A Life in Balance* are Backyard Bar-B-Q Pan Fired Tempeh, Beloved Burritos, Garlic

Spaghetti, Stovetop Beans, and Vegetable Stir Fry with Tofu. The recipe for Mighty-Good Minestrone Soup is also straightforward.

Here's an example of how easy healthy eating can be with my own variation of Meg's recipe for her Beloved Burritos. Canned beans are a fine alternative to cooking them yourself:

1 cup black beans
1 cup pinto beans
1 package of large tortillas: rice will eliminate concerns with gluten
4 cups cooked brown rice (2 cups uncooked)
2 chopped avocados
5 sliced cucumber sour pickles
½ head of lettuce or Napa cabbage thinly sliced
salsa
hummus

Steam or microwave the tortillas for less than a minute, spread them with hummus, add the ingredients, wrap them up, then serve.

SUMMING IT UP

Paying attention to what your child eats can make an enormous difference. He may be eating foods that create a friendly environment for bacteria to grow, inflame his system, or produce allergic reactions that divert his immune system and pose further health risks. The important thing about dietary changes is to just get started. You don't have to do everything all at once, just try to make one change a week. Pick one piece of your child's diet and focus on improving that. Perhaps you decide to eliminate all soft drinks one week and ice cream the next. Or you may decide to experiment with eliminating dairy products from your home. In the journal you'll be creating under chapter 8, "Working Together with the Doctor" you'll be able to easily track whether the changes are producing an effect. Be patient. Dietary changes may take a few weeks to produce results as the system slowly clears itself.

By taking the steps mentioned in this chapter, you will be placing your child in a much better position to harness the strength of the immune system. The human body has a remarkable ability to heal; help your child tap into its miraculous power.

BIG IDEAS FROM CHAPTER SIX

❑ There are three goals when it comes to feeding your PANDAS child:
    starve the bacteria
    reduce inflammation
    boost the immune system.
❑ The vast majority of the immune system resides in the intestinal tract, so keeping the intestinal tract healthy is crucial to having a healthy immune system.
❑ Bacteria thrive on sugar.
❑ Allergies cause inflammation.
❑ Your child may be having an allergic reaction to food that you do not even know about.
❑ Probiotics help to prevent your child from developing a leaky gut.
❑ Your child should eat nutrient-dense foods as often as possible.

III FACILITATING TREATMENT

Assembling the Treatment Team of Doctors and Other Clinicians

7

Dear Beth,
My child has been diagnosed for a year with OCD. The doctor finally agreed to run a blood test and the strep titer came back at 1000. The doctor says it's a coincidence. I've given him your book and lots of articles, but he still doesn't believe in PANDAS. Can you point me to the latest research so I can convince him?
High Titer Mom

Dear High Titer Mom,
I think a better use of your time would be to find a new doctor, one who is willing to recognize PANDAS and treat it. The more time that passes without treatment, the more severe the symptoms may become.
Beth

PANDAS is believed to be caused by a systemic aberration: strep antibodies cross the blood-brain barrier, enter the brain, and attack the basal ganglia. Think of it as walking a path through the snow. The first time it's tough to trudge a path through the snow from the house to the shed. The second time it's not as hard. By the time you've walked that path twenty times, it's easy. Similarly, the first time PANDAS strikes, it forges new pathways in the brain. Over time, everything happens more quickly, and the behavioral exacerbations grow steadily worse with each subsequent episode of PANDAS. Failing to intervene early or treat properly risks that the condition may become

FACT: Each time PANDAS strikes and causes behaviors to flare it is called a behavioral exacerbation.

chronic. This is why it's important to make sure that your child receives prompt appropriate treatment. Once you believe PANDAS is a likely factor in your child's illness, you will need to assemble a treatment team made up of members who are willing to work with you and with each other.

This chapter is about choosing the right people.

The Members of the Treatment Team

When I refer to the *treatment team*, I am including the entire group of doctors and therapists who will become involved in your child's life. Each member has different qualifications and brings a different perspective to the case. It is important for you to understand the differences between the training, qualifications, and perspectives of those professionals who may become involved. You need to understand what each person is capable of providing for you and why each may approach your situation differently. If you do not understand those differences, you will expect

FACT:

Physicians can prescribe medication. Physician assistants (PAs) and nurse practitioners (NPs) can also prescribe in certain defined circumstances.

things from them that are not consistent with what they can offer. When you understand what each has to offer, you will be able to ask the right person for the right information and help speed recovery.

Whenever I use the word *doctor* in this book, I am referring to a physician. A physician is able to prescribe medication and holds a medical degree (MD) or a doctor of osteopathy (DO). *Physician assistants* and *nurse practitioners*, each of whom can prescribe medication, work directly under the supervision of or by an agreement with a physician (although in some states nurse practitioners can own their own practice). Therefore, while the physician assistant or nurse practitioner may be prescribing medication and seeing your child regularly, the physician is the one ultimately responsible for the child's treatment. The services of a physician assistant and/or nurse practitioner will generally fall under my use of the word doctor unless I mention otherwise.

When I am referring to a psychologist or other professional who works with the child in a behavioral capacity, I may call that person a therapist. A therapist does not have the qualifications needed to prescribe medication. It's a common error to confuse psychiatrists (who are physicians) with psychologists. A psychologist holds a master's degree (MA) or a doctorate (PhD). A psychologist is trained to

FACT:
A psychologist offers therapy, but cannot prescribe medication.

observe, assess, and modify human behavior through the application of various approaches and principles. A clinical psychologist will usually be the professional who provides the day-to-day cognitive and developmental help your child will need to conquer behaviors. A psychologist might also be involved in the initial assessment or "work up" of your child's disorder. Remember though, most psychologists— like most doctors—are not well versed in PANDAS, so you may be the one suggesting the possibility of the diagnosis.

Social workers may hold a bachelor, master's or doctorate degree. Social workers study family or societal systems. Their training does not usually include consideration of medical explanations for behavioral problems. There are primarily two settings where social workers may become involved in your situation: at the hospital and at school. If your child ends up at the hospital through an emergency room admission for crisis behaviors, the social worker on staff will probably meet with you. Hospital social workers are often trying to determine if there are issues of abuse or neglect in the home that require referral to the appropriate state agency. Schools often have social workers on staff, too. They may hold full-time or part-time positions and sometimes serve a number of schools within a particular district. They are trained to look for familial problems as an explanation of what is going on with your child, so that will be their focus. It will be rare for a social worker to remain as part of the ongoing treatment team for your child, unless social services are already in place in your home.

Counselors may hold a bachelor's degree or have no formal education. Absent unusual circumstances, a counselor generally will not have the expertise needed to work with a PANDAS child. Therefore, if you are referred to a counselor, carefully ascertain his or her credentials.

During a presentation for a group of students pursuing master's degrees in social work, I told them the story of a family I was working with at the time. The family's ten-year-old daughter had been misdiagnosed for six years with various psychiatric conditions before her mom found *Saving Sammy*, located the right doctor, and subsequently confirmed the child had PANDAS. I mentioned all the little girl's behaviors and explained the damage caused by the disorder and by the psychotropic medications she'd been erroneously prescribed for years. The toll had left her unable to get to school. In spite of her parents' extraordinary efforts over the years, school personnel relentlessly blamed them for not trying hard enough to get her there. Finally with the appropriate diagnosis, coupled with my legal skills and knowledge of the disorder, we secured the educational help she needed. At the conclusion of my presentation, one of women in the audience approached me. Distraught, she said she was a social worker for a local school system, working with a family whose son sounded remarkably similar to that little girl. She and the rest of the school team had been blaming the parents. She said she was going to call the family that afternoon to suggest they look into PANDAS. As well meaning as this social worker had been, her training had simply never led her to consider the possibility that the parents were trying as hard as they could, and that an infection might be the root cause of the problem.

Knowing Yourself

You love your child and would do anything if it would help. The fact that you are reading this book shows how deeply you care. I would have done a back flip off Mount Kilimanjaro if I thought it would have helped Sammy, and I am willing to bet that you would do the same for your child, too. Still there is that lingering doubt about whether we caused this. We examine every aspect of our lives and hound ourselves with the questions. Is this my fault? Did the new baby take too much time away from him? Is it because she's an only child? Am I impatient? Should I have been willing to let him play longer at the park, or let more friends come to play? Is it because of the divorce? Did I let him stay up too late at night? Was it that glass of wine I had when I was pregnant? Did I feed him enough vegetables? Was it too many late nights at the office? Is it the stress of my new job? Did I turn her into a neat freak by making her clean up her toys? Did she stop eating because I mentioned that my friend's daughter was putting on weight? Is he pulling his hair out because I kept telling him it was too long? Is it something about this new house? Are my parenting skills really as bad as the school thinks they are?

Believe me when I say this: I get it. I've been there. Now believe me when I say this: it's not your fault.

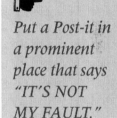

Put a Post-it in a prominent place that says "IT'S NOT MY FAULT."

All the guilt and relentless self-doubt will only gum up the works, so you have to stop beating yourself up and let it go. Whether it's PANDAS or a mental health ailment unrelated to strep, it isn't your fault. Certainly there are children who are so neglected and abused by their caregivers that they end up with neuropsychological damage. Those cases are very few, and something tells me that you are not one of those caregivers because you're taking the time to read this book. If you need to stick Post-its all over the house saying, "IT'S NOT MY FAULT," do it. Stop talking to anyone who tells you differently. When they call, tell them someone's at the door and you have to go. If you see them in person, get away quickly. You don't need poisonous people in your life. I call them "time wasters." You don't have time for them because you are going to be really busy finding the right treatment providers for your child and then managing his care. You are the CEO of your very ill child's life and running interference with unhelpful people is not part of your job description.

FACT: You know your child better than anyone else, and you are the person who cares the most.

Knowing Your Child

You will be your child's primary advocate. Treatment will be provided primarily based upon the information you provide. You know your child better than anyone else, and you are the person who cares the most. If you feel something is "off," or if the information you are given by treatment providers doesn't feel right, you need to trust your instincts. There isn't anyone who knows your child better than you: not a relative, not a teacher, not a neighbor or doctor. It doesn't matter if they hold an advanced degree and you didn't graduate from high school. The person who holds the key to your child's recovery is you. Your child is a vulnerable little soul who has been entrusted to you. What will shape your child's life is your advocacy and care. The information you are able to provide will be invaluable to your child's treatment. There will be times when the information you receive is complicated and the path isn't clear, but you will be there for your child at every step of the way. You are the person who knows if there was a change in the pattern of his behaviors. The teachers don't know that. You do because you are the person who has raised him. You know if the therapy is working because you are with him more than any other observer. You can tell whether it's having an impact. You know how he is responding to medication. You live with him and observe him constantly, not just in an office for a brief appointment when he might hold it together and then let loose at home. If the medication is not working, you are the person who knows it. You are the most important person in your child's life.

Finding the Right Treatment Members

You are assembling a team you may be working with for quite a while. Be a careful manager. Take your time and ask questions before making decisions about who will be on the team.

PANDAS requires tireless tracking and an open exchange of information between all the key players. Of all the adults involved in making sure your child recovers, you are the one who matters most. The treatment team providers should be there to guide and support you, not make you feel deficient. Your team needs members that not only have the information you need, but are willing to hear what you have to say, respect your opinions, include you in decisions, explain the treatment plan to you understandably, and clearly answer your questions. So the providers need to be persons with whom you feel comfortable. This means that when you speak with them, you need to feel they are truly hearing your concerns and responding to your questions. If you don't feel that is happening, then they are not the right choices for the team. Think of this as a sports team with you as the manager. You couldn't have coaches and players unwilling to listen or effectively respond. Of course you are responsible for communicating clearly, but if you are doing your best and simply cannot "connect" with someone, then that person may not be the best choice for your team.

As you meet with a provider for the first time, the questions you should ask yourself are:

❑ Do you feel the two of you can build a rapport?
❑ Will you feel comfortable bringing your concerns and fears to this person or do you feel intimidated?
❑ Is the person patient with you or are you being rushed?
❑ Can he or she explain things to you in such a way that you understand what is being said?

While these considerations may run through your mind during the first visit that you have with any provider, PANDAS is unique. Chemistry with your provider might be less important for some conditions. If you need a knee replacement, you may simply want the surgeon who will do the best procedure. It's a relationship with a defined endpoint, but you, your child, and your PANDAS provider will probably all be involved for quite some time. Choosing members of this team goes beyond assessing whether the candidate has the skills you need. Treatment providers have personalities just as we all do. The doctor who your best friend thinks is terrific, might not be the right one for you. If you and a doctor do not connect, it doesn't mean that there is something wrong with either of you. It just might not be the right fit and that's important here. You will be juggling many different and crucial considerations, so making sure each

Each member will bring something different to the team; be able to identify what each person adds and how that person will help you.

member of your team is a good fit may determine how quickly your child responds and recovers.

On the other hand, it's rare that one person will offer everything you need. A physician may have the information and treatment protocol you need, while the therapist may be your best "go-to" person. The key is to view this as a team effort with each member bringing something you need. A great catcher may not hit the most home runs, but you need both types of players on the team. Can you put your choices together into a team that will work well for you and your child?

An additional point to consider is whether your potential team members have worked together before. If they have, this will help save time. So if you have found the physician you believe is the right choice and that physician recommends a therapist (or vice versa), you should seriously consider that recommendation.

Beyond personal rapport, there are baseline standards to help you decide whether a provider should be on your team. If the provider doesn't meet the standards, you need to make a different choice. Or if it seems as time goes on that your choice might not have been the best, then you will need to make a change. Let's discuss the baselines that will help you make good choices. Keep in mind that there are many doctors at world famous institutions who do not believe PANDAS, so don't necessarily be swayed by credentials.

Basic Requirements for Members of Your Treatment Team

Dear Beth,

I read your heartwarming story about Sammy. I also have a son who suffers from OCD. His symptoms started between ten and eleven years old. I went in to see our family doctor last week and asked for a strep type A blood test. She said even if the test came back positive she would not be able to treat it, so she wouldn't order the test. Does that make sense?

Stunned

Dear Stunned,

No, it does not make sense that a doctor would not want to have as much relevant information about a patient as possible. My suggestion is that you try to find a physician who is open to the diagnosis. It's the personality you're looking for . . . someone intelligent and open-minded who is not threatened by new theories in medicine. Until then, for a list of walk-in labs—no doctor's order is needed—visit anylabtestnow.com.

Beth

Choosing a Physician. The first and probably most important decision will be to choose the right physician. When it comes to PANDAS, physicians fall into three groups.

The first group is the doctors who do not believe that PANDAS exists. There is no point wasting time with a doctor who is part of that group. At the opposite end of the spectrum is a group of doctors who are experienced in treating the disorder. Working with an experienced physician will be ideal, but there are only a few hundred in the country. One may not be located near you or the in-network limitations of your insurance policy may preclude access. Therefore, your next best choice will be to find a doctor who is open to the disorder and wants to help. What these doctors all have in common is that they know medicine is always evolving. And when it comes to a sick child, these doctors know it is worth exploring reasonable treatment possibilities. It won't be easy for them to find the information they need because there is no established treatment protocol so you will become an invaluable resource. And because you and the doctor have a good rapport, he or she will rely on you to help track down and provide the necessary information.

> **FACT:**
> *There are basically three groups of doctors when it comes to PANDAS those who...*
> - *already treat it,*
> - *don't believe in it,*
> - *will do their best to help because they know medicine is always changing.*

What the doctor says:

"I have what I believe are logical approaches to PANDAS, but I have not treated enough PANDAS patients to be able to evaluate the results. It's frustrating that there are no treatment guidelines available. I am concerned that it may be another ten or twenty years before the body of mainstream medicine is extensive enough to satisfy the American Academy of Pediatrics, the American Medical Association, or the American Academy of Child and Adolescent Psychiatrists."

Robert Sears, MD, FAAP (Dr. Bob)

Will the doctor obtain and share information? You must choose a doctor who is willing to receive information from you, obtain the needed information, and easily share it with you. At a minimum, if your doctor is not willing to order blood tests, tell you what tests are being ordered, and give you physical copies of the results, then that doctor cannot be on your team. The members of your team need to work with you and openly share information. It's not a game of hide and seek. So if you sense it will be a struggle to obtain information from your doctor, that doctor will not be a good choice for the team.

Is the doctor open to PANDAS? If you are not able to find an experienced doctor, you want to bring a doctor on board who is at least open to PANDAS. It's not hard to tell where a doctor stands. Listen to what the doctor says when you mention PANDAS. In the middle of polishing my manuscript for Saving Sammy, I ended up in the emergency room with appendicitis. Reviewing my history, the surgeon asked me a number of questions including what I did for a living. When I explained about writing my book and PANDAS, Kevin Price, MD, commented, "How could I have attended all of my classes in medical school and never heard about this?" He was genuinely intrigued and wanted to hear more. As he learned more about PANDAS, he started mentioning it to colleagues. Dr. Price is the type of doctor you want on your team: someone intellectually curious who is open to the possibilities of advances in medicine.

If the doctor says, "I don't believe it," it's easy. You know that you need to move on, but it may also be more subtle. If you feel a doctor is merely being polite, pay attention to that feeling. You need a doctor who is truly invested. You need someone who will listen to you and be open to what you have to say. You can spend tremendous amounts of energy trying to convince a reluctant doctor that PANDAS exists, or you can find someone who belongs on your team. I vote for the latter. A physician's willingness to be open to the disorder and learn the best practices for treating it will go far. I'm a lawyer, but I have learned all about PANDAS. A caring physician can certainly do the same.

A word of caution. There are some doctors who list PANDAS as an area of interest on their website or claim to be specialists in the disorder; but their interest is to get you into their office to explain that PANDAS does not exist. This means you must screen carefully by telephone before you set up an appointment. While you would not ordinarily grill a doctor's assistant to make sure the doctor actually treats a particular disorder, you should for PANDAS. The key question you must have answered before seeing a doctor who lists PANDAS as an area of interest is whether the doctor *treats* it. Seeing someone who wants to tell you all the reasons that PANDAS does not exist is not a productive use of your time or money.

*Before you visit any doctor whose website lists PANDAS as an area of interest, make sure that doctor actually **treats** children for PANDAS.*

> *Dear Beth,*
> *I have been tracking my son's PANDAS symptoms since he was five years old. It started when he was throwing his head back and rolling it along his shoulder. My school nurse was the one who told me about PANDAS. By second grade, he had lots of tics and emotional breakdowns that get much worse whenever he has strep. We took him to a famous pediatric neurologist who listed PANDAS on his website. When we mentioned PANDAS, he put up his hand, shut his eyes, and shook his head no. He told us that if it was PANDAS we would be in and out of ERs. Is he right?*
> *Jittery*

Dear Jittery,

The common sense goal should be to treat the children before they are so sick that they need to be hospitalized, not to use the ER as a barometer. Please see a different doctor and make sure the doctor treats PANDAS, not just has theories about it.

Beth

People Who Don't Make the Team. Not everyone gets to make the varsity team and that is true of your PANDAS team, too. If either of these two key questions raise concerns for you about someone you are considering, it may be best to select someone different.

Are you being blamed? One clue that a person should not make the team is if your parenting skills are being identified as the problem. The notion that emotional and mental disorders are caused by poor parenting skills is old school. If you find yourself defending your parental responses to the symptoms of PANDAS, I'd think seriously about whether that person should be a treatment provider. For example, I attended a very concerning grand rounds presentation at a hospital one morning. Grand rounds are short educational seminars offered in particular areas of medicine at teaching hospitals. The doctor, who claimed to be an expert on pediatric OCD, opened by stating that he would not be discussing PANDAS at all, "because it's controversial." I knew we were off to a less than ideal start. Eventually, he showed DVD footage of mothers attempting to soothe their tormented children. I thought they had come up with some effective strategies to respond to the anxiety and torture that their sweet darlings were enduring on a daily basis. He said their actions were causing the disorder to grow worse. Here was an "expert," who wouldn't even mention PANDAS, pronouncing the children's mothers as having deficient parenting skills. Forget making the team; he shouldn't even be invited to tryouts.

> **FACT:**
> *You are frustrated because of your child's behaviors. The behaviors are not being caused by your frustration.*

You and your family are doing your best to manage an incredibly ill child. If you are being criticized rather than being recognized for doing your best to cope, if you feel guilty or ashamed, you need a different provider. Your frustration is not causing your child's behaviors; you're frustrated because of the behaviors. If a treatment provider is unwilling or unable to see that distinction, then he or she will probably miss the PANDAS boat, too, or at least be a reluctant rower. You need to surround yourself with positive, supportive team members who are all going in the same direction.

Is there a disagreement over medication or approach? Your PANDAS child will probably be treated with two different types of medication: antibiotics (for the infection) and psychotropics (for the mental health symptoms). Those medications may be prescribed by up to three different physicians who may all be part of the treatment team: a pediatrician (or family practitioner), a developmental pediatrician, and a psychiatrist. The therapist will not be prescribing, but will want to offer input into what appears to be helping. Everyone has to be able to work together, and you may become the point person responsible for making sure everyone has the information they need. Even if you do not become the hub for direct distribution of information, you always need to know what's happening.

To achieve that, you need to be able to talk openly with all of your child's providers. You need to know why one medicine is being prescribed rather than another. You need to feel comfortable asking questions about the medicine and understanding its intended effect. Otherwise, you may not know what to look for. Your observations about what is working for your child should be the most important information that the team can gather. If the members of the team are not working together, or if one member is not willing to hear what you or another provider have to offer, then that person is not a good choice for the team.

Even more important, you cannot have a member of the team who is an active nonbeliever. If a member of the team causes you to feel defensive or you constantly have to justify the decisions being made, then that person may need to be replaced. There is a difference between caring, thoughtful discourse, and a provider who wants to hold the team back.

I do know of situations where a given treatment provider has not necessarily embraced PANDAS as a diagnosis, but was willing to work with the team. In this situation, the dividing line is whether the reluctant provider is a doctor or therapist. A therapist who is not particularly supportive of antibiotic treatment might remain willing to work on the cognitive behavioral aspects of OCD and leave the infectious piece to others. Ideally, you'd rather have a therapist on board who is supportive, but it might work if the skeptical therapist isn't obstructive. If one of your child's prescribing physicians simply does not believe in PANDAS, I think it will be impossible for that doctor to remain on your child's team. Your pediatrician, for example, may have done a good job in the past with annual checkups and ear infections, but now your PANDAS child has an extremely serious medical condition. If the pediatrician is going to continually question the diagnosis and course of treatment, you will need to find someone new.

> *Dear Beth,*
> *I just wanted to share a "joyous" moment thanks to all of your hard work and the encouragement you have given me and my daughter Ellen. She was one of forty-five children who sang the National Anthem with Kelly Clarkson on Superbowl Sunday. If it weren't for your encouragement, she wouldn't be able to experience this fabulous moment in her life. Her psychologist told me that PANDAS rarely exists and that he thinks Ellen should be off the Augmentin soon. He has really helped her with her anxiety problems, but he doesn't have a clue about PANDAS. I will continue to keep her on it, regardless of what he suggests.*
> *Hugs from me and my precious angel!*
> *Superbowl Mom*

SUMMING IT UP

Part of your job as a PANDAS parent is to assemble a treatment team that can meet your child's needs and work well with you. You should approach this as if you were interviewing candidates for the most important job openings that need to be filled with the best possible people. You want team members who have the information you need or are willing to help you find it. You want to work with people who will share openly with you and will respect your important role. You do not want to choose people who blame you for your child's behaviors or make you feel uncomfortable for whatever the reason may be. Take the time and ask the questions you need to feel comfortable about your choices. These are people you will be working with for a long time on behalf of your child. If you feel that a particular person you speak with may not be the right choice, pay attention to your instinct. There are plenty of smart, open-minded physicians and therapists who want to help heal their patients and will do what they can to achieve that goal. Your goal is to find them.

BIG IDEAS FROM CHAPTER SEVEN

❑ Behavioral exacerbations grow worse with each episode of PANDAS so it's important to find the correct medical care early.

❑ Your child's treatment team needs to be composed of members who are willing to collaborate with you and with each other.

❑ In this book the following terms have the following meanings:

Doctor means a practitioner who is qualified to prescribe medication.

Therapist means a psychologist, social worker, or counselor.

Treatment team members are the entire group of doctors and therapists who are working together with you on behalf of your child.

❑ Your child's behavioral disorder is not your fault.

❑ You know your child better than anyone else, and you care the most.

❑ The information you can offer about your child and the child's response to treatment is crucial to recovery.

❑ If you cannot find an experienced doctor, a doctor's openness to the disorder and willingness to learn is the key.

❑ If your parenting skills are being blamed as the reason for your child's behavior, it is probably best to find a different person for the treatment team.

❑ If there is a fundamental disagreement over medication or approach, it will be difficult for your treatment providers to work well together.

❑ You are the most important member of the treatment team.

Working Together with the Doctor

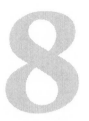

Dear Beth,
I reviewed all of my son's records and was able to pinpoint his first
strep throat infection. I was amazed how much I'd forgotten until I
went back through all the records. Our doctor's appointment went
really well. I think a doctor is willing to pay closer attention when
they see a parent really doing the footwork and having materials
organized and outlined.
Medical Records Mom

Doctors are busy and work very hard. They have many patients, demanding jobs, and families just like the rest of us. Their cars break down. Their plumbers screw up. They even run errands. So you want to make this as easy for them as possible. You want your child to be one of the patients they look forward to seeing because you— as parents and caregivers—have your act reasonably together even when your world is falling apart. The key to working well with your doctor is to be organized and have all the information that your doctor may need to know. This chapter explains the information you should have readily available and how to compile it.

"Be prepared"
should be your motto
for all of your child's
appointments.

Because appointments with PANDAS doctors are at a premium, you want to make the most of your time with the doctor. For that reason, although what you're going through is incredibly sad and difficult, you want to keep your emotions in check during the appointment. This will help keep the focus on medical information. If you need to cry, I recommend saving that for your friends. I cried buckets of tears over Sammy, but I did not cry around his doctors for one reason: it doesn't help with the treatment. Your goal is to get the best possible help for your child and crying might be counterproductive. Plus, if you are sitting there bawling your eyes out, you might forget to mention something important; then you will kick yourself after you leave and perhaps cry even more. That being said, I know sometimes it's tough to keep emotions under control. So let's talk about what you can focus on instead: gathering information. Information is not only less emotional, it will be of enormous help to your child's entire treatment team. Moreover, by empowering yourself with information, you may find yourself crying less.

Meticulous Records

The importance of keeping meticulous records cannot be overemphasized. When you show up at your child's appointment, with your organized records in hand, you will be able to offer information that may make the difference between a clear, steady path to your child's recovery or a difficult, rutty road.

This section covers the record keeping pieces you need to assemble. If you are not comfortable developing your own forms or you want to be able to jump right in and get started, you may want to consider the Tool Kit available on the Products and Services page at savingsammy.net. It includes a package of forms that you can print out and fill in. Many parents have found it helpful.

When you begin to gather the family history, think of yourself as a detective. Follow up on leads and keep asking questions until you're satisfied that the history you've compiled is as complete as possible.

1. Family History: It is crucial that you be prepared to provide an accurate family history. To do this, you need to call members on both sides of your child's family. Take notes and ask questions, particularly about diseases related to infections and autoimmune disorders. The answers may lead to more questions. Here are samples of the general areas you will want to cover:

❑ Is there a family member who struggled with recurrent strep infections?

❑ Did anyone have rheumatic fever?

❑ What about scarlet fever, Sydenham's chorea, nephritis (kidney disease), or rheumatoid arthritis?

❑ Did anyone have tonsils or adenoids removed?

❑ Does anyone in your family have a mental health diagnosis?

❑ Is there is a history of an autoimmune disease on either side of your child's family?

If the answer to any of these is "yes," then you need to dig deeper. Who was affected, when did it occur, and how was it treated? The depth of your information may depend upon who this relative is and when they were sick. Tracking down the history on older relatives will be challenging, but come up with as much information as you can. Ideally, you want to be able to bring to the doctor that family member's name (Sarah), their relationship to your child (great-grandmother), what they had (rheumatic fever), when they had it (late 1940s), and how it was treated (penicillin for many years). While it may be impossible to come up with every piece of information, gather as much as you can.

Make sure your timeline includes important medical information about close family members. If your child started wetting the bed at the same time his sister started battling recurrent ear infections, that's important.

2. Timeline: Your doctor will want to see if there is a connection between the current behaviors and evidence of prior illness. In doctor lingo, this is called a "temporal relationship." There are two people who can take on this responsibility: the doctor or you. It will be far more time and cost efficient if you provide the doctor with the completed timeline rather than having the doctor pour through the pediatric records and put it together. And as you review the records yourself, chances are your memory will be jogged with valuable insights.

Ideally, your goal is to create a timeline that enables the doctor to quickly zero in on the temporal relationship. Think of this as a sidewalk and you are marking the distance you've covered. Your timeline may be relatively simple if you know that your child had strep on a certain date, three days later he started having extreme behaviors that have never stopped, and one month later his titer was through the roof. But if your case isn't that easy—and most are not—I recommend beginning your timeline at least a year before the behavioral problems started. A history from birth will be ideal, at least covering the more important infections, but realistically that is not always possible.

What the doctor says:

"It's not always possible to provide all of this information because 40 percent of strep infections are clinically silent, but making a timeline of the records is important. What I need are the key pieces of information that will enable me to determine whether there is a temporal (time-linked) association between the infection and the onset of abnormal behaviors."

Daniel Geller, MD

You are looking for patterns that may indicate that temporal relationship. You are also looking for earlier subtle or "soft signs" that may have foreshadowed a developing problem.

- ❏ Did she have a problem with wetting the bed every time her sister had strep?
- ❏ Did things first become unbearable when her father was sick with the flu?
- ❏ Was she constantly afflicted with ear infections when she was a baby?
- ❏ Did everyone else get sick with a sore throat, but not her so she was never on antibiotics?

If you are not clear about some of the history, obtain copies of pediatric records to review. You are entitled to these records under the Health Insurance Portability and Accountability Act (HIPAA), but you may have to pay for the copies. You should also call your pharmacy and obtain printouts of the medication prescribed for every family member for the years since the behaviors started. Pharmacies usually have records for the past seven years.

Your child's treatment will only be as good as the information you provide. You are the detective and there will never be a more important case for you to thoroughly research and describe.

Start a daily journal to bullet point behaviors, medications, and eating habits.

3. Daily Journal: Start keeping a daily journal, record your child's behaviors and the medications given each day. This will give you and your treatment team crucial information. I used a dated weekly planner from an office supply store. These also come in daily or monthly choices. There needs to be enough room to write brief notes for each day. You are not writing essays, just bullet points of information. At the very top of each day, for quick reference, you should write down the medication your child received that day. You should also enter the medication and dosage next to the time slot for when she took it. Track eating habits as well. Jot down what she ate and when she ate it. For easy reference, highlight what you feel are the most significant entries.

After a few weeks of tracking, you will be able to see patterns. You may discover that she does better when she takes the medicine at certain times of day or stays away from certain kinds of food. You do not need to write volumes, just brief notes.

Mark an arrow in the left margin beside each day of your journal. Up for a good day, down for a bad day, and horizontal if no swing either way. This will help you quickly track the overall pattern of how your child is doing.

I think it's helpful to mark an arrow in the left margin beside each day. For a good day, the arrow points up. For a bad day, it points down. A horizontal arrow means no particular swing either way. This provides an easy way to get a quick overview of your child's daily progress. When Sammy was sick, this approach was comforting because while there were bad days during his recovery, I could easily see that the good days always returned. Otherwise, that clear indication of recovery might have been lost in my hundreds of short notes.

When you sit down at the appointment with your child's doctor, and you have your journal in hand, you will be able to provide a wealth of information.

A sample journal page might look like this:

FEBRUARY 28
7:00 am *750 mg Amoxicillin*
8:00 am *cereal, ½ hr compulsions*
11:00 am *blueberries and soy yogurt, more compulsions*
12:00 pm *probiotics*
12:30 pm *lunch—miso soup, rice crackers, and bean salad*
1:30 pm *watching television quietly*
2:30 pm *hopping and neck jerking for 10 minutes*
3:00 pm *television again*
4:00 pm *snack, said, "it hurts." crying*
6:00 pm *dinner—chicken, brown rice, broccoli*
7:00 pm *750 mg Amoxicillin*
8:00 pm *resting quietly*
9:00 pm *asleep*

4. Blood Test Chart:

Dear Beth,
I've been charting my child's blood tests for eighteen months and now her strep titer is the highest it's ever been: 860. Her mood swings, joint pains, and shaking have become out of control. The doctors give her drugs that basically tranquilize her. They tell me she could just possess a high titer. They won't even try a high dosage of antibiotics. I've read everything, and I know in my heart that she has PANDAS, but the place I've taken her is a famous clinic. What would you do?
Indecisive in Indianapolis

Dear Indecisive,
I'd take her somewhere else. No one just happens to have that high a titer coupled with all those symptoms. The clinic may be famous, but in this case they're giving you the wrong information.
Beth

Your doctor should be ordering blood tests roughly once every two or three months for tracking purposes. Titers are slow to move, so testing more frequently may not prove beneficial. You can weave the blood test results into your daily journal, but I think it is clearer to have a separate chart that tracks the blood results. What you will be looking for is whether the titer is rising or dropping. When you cross reference a rising titer on your blood chart with the entries in your journal, you will most likely see an increase in behaviors. Similarly as the titer drops, behaviors usually improve. Keep the blood test chart simple. On the left write the date and next to it record the titer. Then add a third entry that records the dosages of medication, particularly the prescribed antibiotics. You will then be able to compare your child's titer with the medication to determine whether the infection is responding. If her titer is elevated and it isn't coming down, you will want to discuss with your doctor whether there needs to be a change in dosage or whether a different choice of antibiotic might be best. Next, add a last column noting behaviors. You chart might look like this:

Date	Titer	Medication	Behavior
8/15	titer 800	1000 mg Augmentin XR	anxiety, OCD
10/31	titer 1200	1000 mg Augmentin XR	crisis behaviors
11/1		increased to 2000 mg Augmentin XR	
1/22	titer 400	2000 mg Augmentin XR	mild OCD, mood good

You need to chart blood test results even though the doctor already has copies. First, it will give you a quick reference tool. Second, although your doctor will have the blood results as individual sheets of paper or an electronic record, the doctor will not have cross-referenced the results with medication and behaviors. Flipping through or visually scanning voluminous results from months of blood tests is not the most efficient way to follow what is going on, and making things easy is part of your job. The results you compile will help you and the doctor to easily mark your child's progress and make pivotal decisions regarding your child's future treatment.

Do you remember the graph your pediatrician kept that tracked your child's height and weight beginning at infancy? That graph let you and your doctor easily track whether growth was on target. You want to create a similar tool for tracking your PANDAS child's onset and recovery.

5. Visual Recording:

Dear Beth,
My son was diagnosed with PANDAS about six months ago. He had a great response to antibiotics. Now he is off them, and I can see that the tics are coming back. His bedwetting is getting worse and his mood is more agitated. The doctor wasn't sure if what I described is a flare-up, but I just know it is. The problem is that when we visit the doctor he keeps everything under control, so the doctor never sees it and feels he is doing well. I'm nervous too much time will go by before he's on Augmentin again, but I don't want to overstep the doctor. What would you do?
Tic-ing Time Clock's Mom

Dear TT's mom,
Children can often hold it together for defined periods of time, and it sounds as if that is what your son is doing. Your doctor needs to be able to actually see the behaviors. Can you record the tics and examples of the mood swings so that you can show the doctor what you are concerned about? Perhaps you can then e-mail the clip to the doctor's office.
Beth

One of the most powerful things you can do is to visually record your child's behavior. You've heard the expressions "seeing is believing" and "a picture is worth a thousand words." Those expressions have never been more true than here. It may be difficult to explain your child's behaviors, and some children manage to keep it all under wraps at the doctor's office. Even if you do your best, your most descriptive explanation of your child's complex tic cannot possibly compare with being able to show the doctor exactly what it looks like. In all of our public appearances, nothing has been more compelling than the Before-During-After footage of Sammy that clearly documented the course of his illness and recovery.

> **FACT:**
> *The camera doesn't lie. A visual record of your child's behaviors and improvements will be one of your most powerful pieces of information. Share it carefully so your child will not be embarrassed.*

Use a camera or your smart phone, but record those behaviors. Usually the children don't want to be filmed. They are sick, and they know it. You would not want to be recorded when exhibiting behavioral problems and neither do they. Nonetheless, as much as we always want to be straightforward with our children, recording behaviors will provide vital information for the treatment team, so you have to be creative. I've seen clips taken of children while one parent drove and the other quietly recorded. The children's facial tics and thrashing limb movements are clearly visible as they travel along in their car seats. I personally poked a camera around corners and out windows so that Sammy did not notice me recording. Eventually, as your child recovers, looking back and seeing the progress will not only be comforting, but proof positive that the path you've chosen is working. Be discreet about sharing that footage, though. You don't want your child traumatized by sharing it too widely. By the time we publicly shared footage of Sammy, he was in college and solidly recovered with many years safely between him and his childhood illness.

Getting Ready for the Appointment

1. Telling the Story. A good way to get ready for your appointment is to think about how you would explain to a friend what has happened since you were last together. If this is your first appointment, think over how you would tell your friend about what brought you to this point. In preparing to tell your story, review all of your materials including your family history, timeline, journal, the blood test chart, and the visual recordings. You wouldn't just hand these to a friend and let her figure it out. You'd tell your friend what happened and have the materials on hand in case you needed to refer to them. It should be the same for your appointment. Look everything over a few times, then practice telling your story until you can do it in a clear, concise, chronological manner.

Practice telling your story before your appointment. Pretend you are seeing a friend for the first time in a long time. How would you tell that friend what has happened since you were last together?

2. What to Bring With You. Your records will be your roadmap for making each appointment productive. Bring along *an extra copy of the timeline*, so that you can hand it to the doctor. A discussion of the family history may be a large part of your first appointment. Organize your notes as *bullet points* that you will refer to throughout the appointment. In your bullet points, include all medical history important to the disorder, including what you have learned from family relatives. Developmentally, you need to be able to describe your child before you suspect PANDAS struck and how she has changed. Assuming your child is on medication, you need to have the dates and dosages at your fingertips, so bring an extra copy of the printout from the pharmacy to give the doctor.

Your bullet points might start something like this for a first visit:

- ❑ Toilet trained at twenty-four months
- ❑ Normal development until age seven: friendly, happy, healthy
- ❑ First grade: four strep infections, each treated with amoxicillin for ten days
- ❑ Did well in school until second grade
- ❑ 9/25 - handwriting changed
- ❑ 10/4 - coughing, throat clearing
- ❑ 10/10 - wetting the bed
- ❑ 10/11 - wouldn't leave my side

Plan to leave the doctor with a copy of your timeline, a printout of all medication from the pharmacy, and the names and contact information for all of your child's treatment providers.

Below the bullet points, write down the *questions you want to cover*. Make sure you understand the answers that the doctor gives to your questions. Medical information can be overwhelming. If you don't understand, ask again. This is complicated stuff. It's okay to ask for another explanation because— remember—you are only working with treatment team members who are supportive of you. You don't need to begin with, "I know this is a dumb question, but..." Nothing you are going to ask is dumb because every question you ask is about something that will help your child get better. By preparing your questions in advance, you won't leave and later remember things that you meant to ask. Everything you want to know will be on your list. If something that the doctor says during the visit triggers another question, jot it down as a late add-on at the end of your list.

Bring along the *visual recordings* of your child's behaviors, and a list of *all your child's treatment providers* with their contact information. This list will be kept with your child's records. Although you will probably be the hub in the wheel of providers, the list will make it easy if one provider wants to speak directly with another.

3. Helping Your Child Have a Good Visit. You must bring your child to the visit. Sometimes the children are too sick to actively participate in their appointments. Many won't even acknowledge that they have any symptoms. It may be too painful for them to do so or, in the case of OCD, the "rules" prevent the discussion. Age is a factor and frustration is another possibility. Nonetheless, the doctor needs to physically see the child to do a proper assessment. Sammy had suffered with endless behaviors and ineffective psychiatric care for a full year before he saw Catherine Nicolaides, MD, who diagnosed him with PANDAS. Her initial observation was that he had a tremor, which no one else had noticed. It was a sign of serotonin syndrome, caused by too high a dose of an SSRI. If he hadn't come to the appointment, the doctor would not have spotted the tremor.

What the doctor says:

"Parents sometimes ask if they need to bring their child to the appointment. I always say yes. It's important for me to see the child in person to do a thorough clinical evaluation."

Catherine Nicolaides, MD

For whatever reason, your child may not be much help during the first several visits. By the time a child sees a PANDAS doctor, he may have already seen many doctors who have been unable to help. As hopeless as you feel, it is also devastating for your child. About the only thing Sammy said at our initial appointment with Dr. Nicolaides was, "Face it, Mom, I'm a failure." While it's best not to build expectations, I do think you should talk encouragingly about the visit and the doctor in advance. Age-appropriate statements about why you think this visit might be different may be helpful. You might talk about how you found this doctor, what is different about this doctor, or what you've heard about this doctor from other parents. Your child may not be willing to say much, but he'll hear what you're saying. I would explain that you plan to be your child's voice at the appointment, but that he should feel free to speak up if you say anything incorrectly. Point out that when he feels better, you know he will probably have more to say. You might gently review what you plan to say so that there are no surprises when the child hears you talk with the doctor. You might ask your child if there's anything that he wants you to tell the doctor. If he says, "No," just say, "Okay, let me know if you change your mind." Talking about the upcoming visit will help reduce anxiety.

This is information that you can convey to your child in sound bites over the days leading up to the visit. You already know what the visit will cover because you are thoroughly prepared with your family history, timeline, journal, chart, and visual recordings. You have already thought about how you will explain to the doctor what has happened. All you need to do is present an age-appropriate version to your child.

During the Appointment

Plan to give your doctor a copy of the timeline. Have readily available your bullet point list of behaviors and questions with a pen to check off the items you cover. This will help to make sure you reach all your topics. While the doctor is talking, jot down notes and buzz words as you go along so that you don't forget anything. You will definitely want to refer to those notes later. If you're not sure you understood something correctly, repeat it back. For example, "I want to make sure I understand this, Doctor. She should take one pill in the morning and one at bedtime?" Find out the best way to communicate with this doctor:

- ❑ How quickly will telephone calls be returned?
- ❑ Would the doctor prefer that you leave detailed messages with office staff or speak directly with the doctor?
- ❑ Will the doctor respond to e-mails?
- ❑ Is it helpful to fax information?

It's often helpful to take a family member or friend along as a support person on important medical appointments. There may simply be so much information conveyed that keeping it straight may be challenging. Two sets of ears will be better than one. Another option might be to record the appointment, so you can play it back later to listen. Being free from the burden of taking notes may enable you to follow along more closely. If you do want to use a recorder, check with the doctor in advance just to make sure that he or she doesn't mind.

> *In speaking with your child about PANDAS, you have three goals: relieve anxiety, offer reassurance, and obtain information. If what you know does not further one of those goals, then keep it to yourself.*

Including Your Child in His or Her Treatment

Because your child may be your most valuable source of information on what is working, you will want to include your child in her treatment as is appropriate for her age. Children should always be protected from more concerning information, so the key is to find the right balance between discussing treatment and insulating her. In speaking with your child about her treatment, your goals will be to:

- ❏ relieve anxiety
- ❏ offer reassurance about recovery
- ❏ enlist help obtaining information

If any of the information you have does not further one of those goals, then my suggestion is that you keep it to yourself. For example, suppose blood work shows that your child's titer has risen. Mentioning the rise may only increase her anxiety. You are the one who must decide how much information to share, but err on the side of cushioning your child.

1. Relieve Anxiety. Accomplish this by staying simple: "You have an infection. Sometimes infections cause sore throats. Other times infections cause children to behave differently. You can't help it if you catch a sore throat and you couldn't help this either." Statements like this offer hope and comfort; she knows that none of this is her fault. If you mention that, "lots of children have this," she will not feel so alone. You should not tell your child that her brain is infected or being attacked or anything that sounds so scary. Remember, many PANDAS behaviors thrive on anxiety; you want to reduce it.

2. Offer Reassurance. Even if you foresee a difficult road ahead, stay positive for your child. "I really like this doctor. Now that we know what it is, you will be able to get better." If the child wants to know when she'll be better, say, "The doctor says it may take a while because all kids are different, but now we know how to get started on helping you get well."

3. Enlist the Child's Help. Let your child know that she is an important part of the recovery process with important information to share. Invite her participation by saying, "I always want you to let me know how you feel." PANDAS children know when the symptoms are coming back. They react to strep the way some children react

Carefully monitor your reactions to your child's disclosures. If she tells you something concerning, smile reassuringly and say that all will be well. Then call the doctor to discuss it once the child is out of earshot.

to peanuts; if they are around it, their symptoms return. A PANDAS child might say, "It hurts," or "It's painful," or "It's coming back." You want your child to openly share that information, not hide it, because knowing how your child feels will help you to get her the right treatment. I'd be cautious, though, about telling her when you are changing medications or dosages only because you do not want that information to color her response; you want as little outside influence as possible so you can accurately gauge the effect.

Part of your child's willingness to share information may depend upon your reaction to her disclosures. Even if you are upset by what you hear, smile and say, "Thank you for telling me. I will call the doctor and find out what to do." Whenever possible, you should refrain from having telephone conversations with the doctor in front of your child. When it comes to sick children, discussing the illness in front of them may be too upsetting for everyone involved. In addition, if you become emotional during the conversation it will be best if the child does not see this. You want to win the Academy Award for staying positive and confident in front of your PANDAS child.

Children with mental health ailments and behavioral disorders sometimes hide or "cheek" their pills. Make sure you watch your child swallow every pill until she is well on the way to recovery and understands that taking her medication is part of why she is getting better.

Having your child invested in her recovery means not only that she shares how she is feeling, but eventually assumes responsibility for making sure she takes her medication. You foster good self-care skills and independence in other aspects of your child's life such as eating habits and exercise. If taking medication is part of what keeps your child healthy, you want her actively involved in that, too. Shifting the responsibility for taking medication is a gradual process that depends on the age and health of the child. I started this shift by purchasing a weekly AM-PM pillbox. You can find one at any pharmacy. Then I divided up the medications for each day. In the beginning, I handed Sammy his pills and watched him take every one. As he became better about it and older, I gradually taught him to remember to ask for the pill box. Then he began to remember on his own. Of course, I'd watch him take the pills and prompt him if he forgot; but he slowly became primarily responsible for taking his medication.

Changing Doctors

> *Dear Beth,*
> *I used to think my child's psychiatrist was good. But ever since my pediatrician figured out that PANDAS is causing my child's behaviors, the psychiatrist has been difficult. I think we have to change. How do I do that and what should I tell him?*
> *Need Guidance*

As difficult as it may be, there may come a time when you do need to change doctors or other treatment providers. There are many reasons for deciding to change. Perhaps your child simply is not getting better, so you feel a change is needed. You may have found someone you think is better than your original choice or perhaps the dynamic between you and a team member has shifted. You may no longer feel comfortable asking questions. You may feel intimidated. You may not be satisfied with the answers you are receiving to questions. You may feel that "do no harm," one of the guiding principles of practicing medicine, is being offered as a reason to refrain from taking the actions that you feel are important. For whatever the reason, once you've made the decision, the question is what to do next.

FACT: *Sometimes it's in your child's best interest to change doctors, even though it can be hard to do.*

It's best to be kind when you end any relationship and part of how you handle this will have to do with the nature of your relationship with the doctor. If this is a pediatrician who has been in your child's life for years, you may feel it's important to meet and explain your decision. If it is a relatively new relationship, calling by telephone to inform the office staff may be enough. Keep in mind that, either way, *explaining* your decision and *defending* your decision are two different things. You do not need to defend your decision, and you are also not responsible for how the provider feels about you leaving. Your only actual obligation is to respectfully notify the provider that you are making a change. It will probably be best to have the new provider selected before you inform the original team member that you are making a change.

If you are changing providers, you will need to request that copies of your child's records be transferred to the new provider. Medical records are owned by the provider or facility that prepares them, but ordinarily providers will transfer copies of medical records without charge between one another as a courtesy. There is, however, no requirement that records be furnished for free. If you ever want your own set of records, which can be requested at any time, you will most likely be charged for the copies. Individual states set the maximum fees that can be charged as guided by the Health Insurance Portability and Accountability Act (HIPAA). In general, the charge must be reasonable and based on cost. Many providers and facilities are moving to electronic records, which may make providing copies easier. Sometimes the delay in transferring records can be frustrating. However, if you have followed the advice in this chapter, you will already have all the necessary information for your new provider to move forward. You have your family history, timeline, journal, and blood test chart. You have your visual recordings. And you have a printout of all medications from your pharmacy. You want those medical records transferred, but even without them you should be in good shape to proceed with the new team member.

> **FACT:**
>
> *As a courtesy, providers will usually transfer medical records free of charge to other providers. But if you want your own set of records, which you are always entitled to have, expect to be charged a reasonable amount for those additional copies.*

Dear Beth,

Thanks for reassuring me that it was okay to change doctors. It was hard because we had been with the same pediatrician for a long time. My biggest insecurity was that I would insult the doctor. Parents really need to know it's okay to ask for second opinions and to seek help from other doctors.

Thoughtful Mom

SUMMING IT UP

If you have followed the guidelines in this chapter, you will be placing your child, yourself, and your doctor in the best possible position for effective treatment. You will be helping your doctor because you will be keeping track of all the important information and presenting it in a concise form. This will result in a more efficient appointment where the focus will be on treatment rather than trying to put all the pieces together. Moreover, having the necessary information will help you feel empowered and confident. The result will be a good working relationship with your doctor and an easier course of treatment for your child.

BIG IDEAS FROM CHAPTER EIGHT

❏ Part of your job is to make this as easy as possible for your child's doctor.
❏ Empowering yourself with information will help keep the appointment less emotional, more focused on treatment.
❏ There are five parts to meticulous records:
  Family history
  Timeline, including pharmaceutical records
  Daily journal
  Blood test chart
  Visual recording.
❏ Before the appointment:
  practice telling your child's story concisely and chronologically
  prepare your child.

- ❏ Bring to the appointment:
  - the meticulous records described above
  - bullet point list of your child's developmental milestones and key behavioral changes
  - questions you need answered
  - support person
  - notepad and pen
  - recording device.
- ❏ Include your child in his or her treatment as appropriate for the child's age.
- ❏ Change doctors and other providers when needed.
- ❏ For an easy to fill in package of printable forms, consider the Tool Kit offered on the Products and Services page at savingsammy.net.

Your Child's Providers: Training and Expertise

"Half of what we'll teach you here in medical school will turn out to be wrong, we just don't know which half yet."

A statement often repeated to students in medical school...

Medical students are often reminded throughout their training that medicine changes. It is an ever-evolving body of scientific knowledge, clinical observation, treatment response, and patient interactions. Sometimes, though, as doctors progress in their careers, they tend to rely mostly on what's familiar. When a particular patient's malady appears to be one thing, the doctor may become comfortable with that diagnosis and quickly rule out other possibilities. This is because doctors are trained to think in a specific way. It's called the "differential diagnosis." It means that doctors run a number of potential diagnoses through their thoughts, narrowing down those possibilities to just a few, and then trying to determine which of the few diseases with similar symptoms is the one causing the suffering. It can be a daunting task, and pressure from insurance companies to spend limited time with patients doesn't help.

> **FACT:**
> The "differential diagnosis" is the process of how doctors are trained to think about disease and reach a diagnosis.

Usually the first doctor you bring your child to see when he is ill is the pediatrician or family doctor. You are hoping for answers. You will get them fairly easily when the problem is something as common as an ear infection, but PANDAS is different. Chances are that most doctors won't be thinking about an infection when you describe severe separation anxiety or any other concerning behaviors. The doctor may feel the child needs an evaluation by a mental health specialist because he is concerned that the child is afflicted with a psychiatric or behavioral disorder. Another concern may be that the child's brain or nervous system may be presenting problems. If the doctor does suspect PANDAS and mentions that he or she has heard of it, the doctor may not feel comfortable trying to treat it. The doctor may want you to take your child to a different kind of doctor who may know what to do. For any of these reasons (and more) the doctor may refer you to a specialist. Often the doctor's suggestion or referral is made with little explanation of what these different specialists have to offer. As a result, you may not know what to expect from a different kind of doctor and possibly become frustrated when the doctor's expertise does not match your expectations.

This chapter explains the general training that all doctors receive. It also covers the particular training required for each specialty, and what that special area of medicine is designed to address. By reviewing the doctor's training and focus for each specialty, you may be better able to work with that doctor regarding your child's needs. You will understand why the doctor approaches your child's health from a particular viewpoint and, perhaps, whether that doctor is the right choice from the outset.

Core Training for Doctors

FACT:
All doctors attend four years of medical school and then a residency program at a hospital in their area of interest.

All doctors in the United States must be licensed by the states in which they practice. Licensing requires graduation from an accredited medical school and completion of a residency program. Medical school is a four-year program, and almost all medical schools divide the four years of training into two years of preclinical training and two clinical years. Preclinical years are spent in the classroom studying bodily systems, major diseases, and patient care. The transition from preclinical to clinical years is usually marked by a "white coat ceremony" when the students receive the traditional garb that has been worn by physicians for hundreds of years. During the clinical years, students rotate through the various areas of medicine for periods that vary in length from a week to a few months under the guidance of qualified physicians. There are no "majors" in medical school. It is during clinical rotations that the medical students begin to decide the area of medicine that will be the best fit for them. Upon completing medical school, the graduates apply to residency programs for the specialty they want to practice. The minimum requirement for licensing is a residency program of two years but programs are often longer. Accredited residency programs are offered at teaching hospitals throughout the United States. The graduates are matched based on the needs of the hospitals and the qualifications of the graduates.

Doctors spend their residency years working long hours, treating very sick patients, and learning from more experienced physicians. Residency is a grueling experience. Upon completion of a residency, the doctor applies for licensing in the state where he or she wants to practice. Having a state medical license, however, does not certify that the doctor is necessarily qualified to practice in any particular area of medicine. The gold standard for qualification in a particular specialty is board certification, and it is required by most hospitals and insurance companies. Board certification requires rigorous testing, assessments through peer reviews, continuing education, and periodic testing to maintain the certification. To be board certified, a doctor must have earned an undergraduate degree, earned an MD or DO degree from a qualified medical school, and completed three to five years of full-time experience as a resident in an accredited program.

> *FACT:*
> *Board certification indicates that a doctor has passed and complied with additional exams, assessments, and educational requirements in a particular area of medicine.*

Doctors may further choose to complete fellowships in a particular area of medicine. A fellowship is a two- or three-year post-residency program that offers the physician an opportunity to develop a more targeted expertise. As with residencies, fellowships are offered at university hospitals and medical centers. For example, a psychiatrist might take a fellowship in substance abuse or a pediatrician might take a fellowship in developmental pediatrics. Another relevant area

FACT:
A fellowship program offers a doctor further training in a narrower area of medicine.

for PANDAS where fellowships are offered is neuropsychopharmacology. Neuropsychopharmacology is an interdisciplinary science involving the brain and how medications affect it. A neuropsychophamacologist, however, might be a PhD rather than an MD or DO. Many in the field have a PhD in, for example, molecular biology or neuroscience.

Sometimes your pediatrician or family doctor will refer you to one of the specialists listed below because they truly don't know what else to do. The following list will provide you with an easy reference tool for understanding the type of doctor to whom you have been referred. Even though a doctor's area of expertise, training, and credentials appear on point, you must still screen carefully before the appointment. For example, while you might think infectious disease doctors will know all about PANDAS (because it is triggered by an infection), many do not and can be quite difficult about the diagnosis.

Physician Specialists

Allergy and Immunology. Allergy and immunology is concerned with the prevention, diagnosis, and treatment of problems with the human immune system. Allergy and immunology is a subspecialty of *internal medicine*. Internists are specially trained to solve puzzling diagnostic problems. Internal medicine focuses on adult diseases and includes all areas of a patient's health (but not pediatrics or obstetrics). Internal medicine includes more in-depth training and patient care in a hospital setting and acute care than,

FACT:
Allergists and immunologists treat autoimmune diseases and immunodeficiencies.

for example, family practice. After medical school, a doctor who wants to practice allergy and immunology first completes the three-year residency and becomes board certified in internal medicine. Then for two more years, the doctor will study conditions specific to the human immune system. A doctor who practices allergy and immunology treats diseases associated with autoimmune responses and symptoms of disorders caused by immunodeficiency. PANDAS encompasses both of those areas.

Developmental Pediatricians. Developmental pediatricians (sometimes called behavioral pediatricians) focus on children who have developmental, learning, or behavioral difficulties. Developmental pediatricians usually do not typically treat physical ailments of children, although they have the qualifications to do so. While your regular pediatrician will continue to do well child checks, administer vaccines, and treat ear infections, your developmental pediatrician may be a better choice to treat behavioral and mental health disorders. After medical school, a developmental pediatrician completes a three-year residency in pediatrics, then completes a subspecialty training in developmental-behavioral pediatrics.

> *FACT:*
> *Developmental*
> *pediatricians*
> *specialize in*
> *children with*
> *developmental,*
> *learning, or*
> *behavioral*
> *difficulties.*

They treat children with the full range of disorders associated with PANDAS (OCD, tics, Tourette's, ADHD, etc.) and may have the expertise to treat PANDAS itself.

Emergency. Emergency room (ER) doctors focus on emergent or acute medical care of patients who need immediate medical attention due to trauma, accident, or a major medical event. After medical school, an ER doctor completes a residency of three to four years. If your child becomes out of control and ends up in the emergency room due to a PANDAS episode, an ER doctor's goal will be to help stabilize your child and make recommendations regarding further steps to take. From the emergency room,

> *FACT:*
> *Emergency*
> *doctors are*
> *primarily*
> *trained to*
> *handle physical*
> *traumas.*

your child may be released home or sent to a crisis unit or referred for further hospitalization.

Ear, Nose & Throat (ENT). Commonly known as ENTs, the formal name is otolaryngologist. ENTs specialize in the diagnosis and treatment of disorders affecting the ear, nose, and throat. After

FACT:
An ENT may become involved if there is a decision to remove your child's tonsils or adenoids.

medical school, an ENT doctor completes a five-year residency. They perform medical procedures like tonsillectomies. Because strep hides in the tonsils, some doctors and parents feel that a tonsillectomy may help a PANDAS patient.

Family Medicine. Family practice doctors focus on treating the whole person through all stages of life. After medical school, a family practice doctor completes a residency of three years, rotating through internal medicine, pediatrics, obstetrics-gynecology, psychiatry, and geriatrics. Family practice doctors and pediatricians are in a unique position to help your children if they recognize the signs of PANDAS in its beginning stages. Early intervention with antibiotics may prevent the disorder from becoming chronic.

Dear Beth,
Last week my five-year-old daughter suddenly started moving her arms at the elbow, like flapping wings. Her dad was diagnosed with strep last week. My daughter's throat never hurt, but she cried more than normal and had other behavior changes such as repeating words and spinning. Her strep test came back positive this morning. Thank you for helping us. Because of your work and your son, we knew what to look for and found it in six days. Thank you!
Caught It Early

Immunologist. see Allergy and Immunology.

FACT:
Most infectious disease doctors do not treat PANDAS.

Infectious Disease or Pediatric Infectious Disease. ID specialists have expertise in infections of the sinuses, heart, brain, lungs, urinary tract, bowel, bones, and pelvic organs. Their extensive training focuses on all kinds of infections, including those caused by bacteria, viruses, fungi, and parasites. Most infectious disease doctors are hospital based. Infectious disease is a subspecialty of internal medicine. After medical school, an ID doctor first completes the requirements to become an internist, including a three-year residency in internal medicine. As an internist, the doctor then completes an additional fellowship training program of two or three years in infectious disease. Along with that specialized knowledge comes a particular insight into the use of antibiotics and their potential adverse effects. ID specialists also have additional training in immunology (how the body fights infection), epidemiology (how infections spread), and infection control. Some infectious disease doctors may choose to sub-specialize in a particular disease such as HIV/AIDS. As a group, ID doctors appear rather stubborn about accepting PANDAS as a diagnosis and are not supportive of the long-term antibiotic treatment that is required for many PANDAS patients to recover. However, an ID doctor may be your best choice for treating a strep carrier in your family.

Internist. see Allergy and Immunology.

Neurologist or Pediatric Neurologist. Neurologists focus on the diagnosis, treatment, and prevention of diseases, disorders, and conditions of the brain and nervous systems. Neurology is a subspecialty of internal medicine, which is described under Allergy and Immunology above. After medical school, a neurologist first completes a one-year internship in either internal medicine or medicine/surgery and then three years of specialty training in an accredited neurology residency program. Neurologists comprise the leading group of nonbelievers in the country.

FACT: Many neurologists do not believe in PANDAS.

Pediatrician. Pediatricians specialize in the care of children. After medical school, they spend three years as residents in pediatrics taking care of very sick children before entering private practice. Pediatricians are trained and experienced in the physical, mental, emotional, and social development of children and youth. A pediatrician is probably

FACT:
A knowledgeable pediatrician who intervenes early can help prevent PANDAS from becoming chronic.

the first doctor you will turn to when your child acts out behaviorally. A pediatrician who recognizes the signs of PANDAS and intervenes early with antibiotics may avert what could otherwise become a chronic condition.

> Dear Beth,
> A friend watched you and Sammy on television and sent me a link to your website. This tipped me off that maybe my daughter's sudden "strange behavior" wasn't OCD. I took her to the doctor today and low and behold she has strep throat and is now on amoxicillin. Her doctor thought I was nuts. Thank you!
> Not Nuts

Psychiatrist. Child psychiatrists treat mental and emotional disorders in children. After medical school, they complete a four-year residency in psychiatry working with children and adolescents.

FACT:
Child psychiatrists are among the foremost PANDAS researchers in the country.

During the residency, they complete rotations in primary care, neurology, and inpatient psychiatry, as well as electives in substance abuse, psychopharmacology, and other studies. They may also participate in conducting research. Following residency, a child psychiatrist may choose to complete a two-year fellowship or subspecialty program in major psychiatric issues that afflict children. Many psychiatrists are primarily concerned with medication management as opposed to therapeutic behavioral intervention. While they often prescribe psychotropic medications, it is less common for them to prescribe antibiotics.

Rheumatologist. Rheumatologists treat patients with autoimmune diseases and patients who have diseases affecting their joints. Rheumatology is a subspecialty of internal medicine. After medical school a rheumatologist first completes the requirements

to become an internist, including three
years of internal medicine residency.
After residency, the rheumatologist
completes fellowship training in a two-
year clinical program. PANDAS is an
autoimmune disease.

FACT:
Rheumatologists treat
autoimmune diseases
and joint pain.

Others Prescribing Healthcare Professionals

Naturopath. Naturopathic doctors (NDs) focus on holistic, proactive
prevention, diagnosis, and treatment. NDs are trained to utilize
prescription drugs, although the emphasis
of naturopathic medicine is the use of
nature's healing agents. NDs have graduated
with a four-year college degree and then
attend a four-year naturopathic medical
school. In addition to the basic sciences,
NDs study clinical nutrition, acupuncture,
homeopathic medicine, botanical medicine,

FACT:
Naturopaths are
only licensed to
practice medicine
in sixteen states.

psychology, and counseling (to encourage people to make lifestyle
changes in support of their personal health). NDs are able to prescribe
medication. Only sixteen states currently license NDs to practice. If
you choose to see an ND, please keep in mind that it is unlikely your
PANDAS child will heal without antibiotic treatment.

Nurse Practitioner. Nurse practitioners (NPs) have graduated with
a college degree from a four-year nursing program, obtained licensing
as an RN, and then completed a master's degree program specific
to a specialty they choose. The program's
requirements include completing a certain
number of clinical hours. The required
hours vary depending upon the program,
the type of NP practice, and state regulatory
requirements, but the current minimum
clinical requirement is five hundred hours.
NPs are able to prescribe medications. A
psychiatric/mental health nurse practitioner
(PMHNP) concentrates on mental health
patients. In about twenty states, PMHNPs

FACT:
Nurse practitioners
and physician
assistants are
permitted to
prescribe medicine
in certain defined
circumstances.

may own their own practices. In other states, the PMHNP must have a collaborative relationship with a physician.

Physician Assistant. Physician assistants (PAs) are health-care professionals who are authorized by the state to practice medicine as part of a team with physicians. PAs conduct physical exams, obtain medical histories, diagnose and treat illnesses, order and interpret tests, counsel on preventive health care, assist in surgery, and prescribe medications. Most PAs have earned a four year-college degree and have about three years of health care experience before entering a two-year PA program. In certain PA programs, the candidates attend first-year classes together with the physician candidates. To practice, a PA must pass the physician assistant national certifying exam and will then be identified with PA-C following his or her name.

Therapists

Behavioral intervention and skill building for children afflicted with PANDAS will probably be provided by a psychologist. As with other professionals, a thorough understanding of the disorder is needed to be successful with your child. None of the professionals listed in this section are authorized to prescribe medication. Each of them must be licensed pursuant to the applicable requirements of the state in which they offer services.

FACT:
A psychologist will most likely be the professional who works with your child on cognitive behavioral therapy. Psychologists are not permitted to prescribe medication.

Psychologist. A psychologist holds a master's degree (MA) or a doctorate (PhD). This means the psychologist has graduated from a four-year college and complied with the requirements to obtain the advanced degree. Usually this requires one or two years of additional education after college. An appropriately trained psychologist may provide the day-to-day cognitive and developmental help your child will need because psychologists are skilled in applying psychological principles to modify behavior. A psychologist might also be involved in the initial assessment or "workup" of your child's disorder. Psychologists are sometimes confused with psychiatrists, so it is important to know the distinction.

Social Worker. A social worker may hold a bachelor's, master's, or doctorate. Social workers are often on staff at hospitals and schools. Social workers become involved when there are concerns about abuse or neglect. It will be rare for a social worker to remain as part of the ongoing treatment team for your child unless social services are already in place in your home for another reason.

Counselor. A counselor may hold a bachelor's degree or no formal education. Absent unusual circumstances, a counselor generally would not have the expertise needed to work with a PANDAS child.

SUMMING IT UP

Knowing the expertise of the doctor you are taking your child to see may help you frame your questions. Choosing a therapist is equally important. By becoming familiar with the extent of each professional's education and training you will have a better understanding of that person's approach to your child's health. It will help you be a better advocate.

BIG IDEAS FROM CHAPTER NINE

- ❏ All doctors must be licensed by the state where they practice medicine.
- ❏ A "resident" is a medical school graduate who is at a teaching hospital, learning the hands-on practice of medicine in the specialty he or she has chosen.
- ❏ State licensing requires graduation from a four-year accredited medical school and completion of a minimum two-year residency program (most programs are longer).
- ❏ Board certification signifies compliance with the applicable conditions established for practicing in a particular area of medicine.
- ❏ A "fellowship" is a post-residency program completed by a doctor who wants to gain more expertise in a subspecialty.

IV THINGS TO KNOW ON THE ROAD TO RECOVERY

Recovery and Backslides

10

Dear Beth,
I just wanted to update you...I went to the doctor with my daughter four days ago, and they finally agreed to put her on Augmentin XR...Thanks isn't a big enough word for me to tell you...your encouragement got me across the threshold. It's been only four days and she has so much more energy...her sweet personality and smile is coming back...such a huge difference! Blessings and thanks to you!
My Darling Daughter's Coming Back

There is no one path to recovery. It happens slowly, with patience, diligence, unwavering commitment, determination, and courage. You can offer all of those qualities. Your child will need to chip in with his own determination and courage, but you must contribute the lion's share. Once the pieces are in place—you've found the right doctor, the disorder is correctly diagnosed, the medication is prescribed, and you're satisfied that you've assembled a strong treatment team—the work begins again. This is the time to make sure your child remains firmly pointed toward full recovery.

This chapter will describe the wave pattern most PANDAS children experience on the way to recovery. It will take you through a series of the possible reasons why there may be backslides along the way. At the end of the chapter is one family's story of how they solved the mystery of what was causing their child's backslide.

Staying Positive

A good part of your personal work during recovery will be to stay positive. Unless you are one of the fortunate few who recognized

FACT:
What your child needs to hear is that all will be well, regardless of how you feel at any particular moment.

PANDAS immediately in your child, the road back will be slow and bumpy. If you expect to meet a few stumbling blocks along the way, it will not be so devastating when you hit one. Most important, you must not let your child know how upset you are if recovery is not progressing as smoothly and quickly as you hoped. No matter how much you worry, wonder if she'll ever get better, shed tears, or doubt full recovery, you must work hard to be sure your child only perceives your complete confidence that this will eventually be over. What your child needs to hear is a consistent message of recovery even when the odds seem overwhelming. Each backslide must be, "A slip. It will get better." The sentences that must become part of your daily spoken dialogue are: *You are going to get well. We will figure this out. Other children have recovered from this and so will you. You and I and the doctor are all working on this together. It's just taking longer than we thought.* These must become your mantra. As reported by research described in chapter 15, stress may play a role in opening the blood-brain barrier, so doing everything you can to reduce your child's anxiety is crucial.

How Long Will It Take?

There is no formula for how long recovery will take. From canvassing the many e-mails I've received, if the children have PANDAS and are treated correctly, you may see an initial response within days. The response may be subtle, but you can tell things are better. It may be a slight shift in attitude, a lessening of intensity around certain behaviors, or a willingness to do something that the child has not done for quite some time. The subtle shift lets you know that you're on the right path. It's a good sign—embrace it! True, it may be many months before you finally have your child completely back, but your hard work is paying off and you're heading in the right direction. Remember, with PANDAS you are working on two fronts: battling an infection and healing the immune system. You can support that process with medication and nutrition, but only time will change the way those two interact.

What If There's a Backslide?

When the behaviors flare up again, the questions are how serious it is and whether you need to intervene. Blips and stumbles can be shrugged off. But if your child is consistently losing previous gains—it's called decompensating—there needs to be quick intervention. It's a sign that something is amiss and needs to be addressed quickly. Knowing the difference between a slip and a major nosedive is a skill that you will develop over time by carefully watching your child and relying on your instincts. Often, there is a wave pattern to recovery with PANDAS. Behaviorally the children do better, regress, rally, and slide back again before showing more signs of improvement. I compare it to a baby who is learning to walk. They

> **FACT:** *"Decompensating" is the term used by mental health professionals to describe when a child is consistently losing the gains he has made.*

fall a lot; that's why we call them toddlers. Your child will fall, too, but the general pattern should be progress. Knowing the difference between a pattern of "two steps forward, one step back" and the signs of major deterioration is a talent you will master. Initially, you will rely on tracking through the notes in your journal. Eventually, you will be able to spot it immediately. If your child goes outside to play one day, but stays inside the next, there's no cause for concern. If it becomes a pattern, though, you need to take quick action. There is a difference between a brief regression to old habits and a solid return to past patterns. If your child had been responding, but has now deteriorated into major regressions such as mood swings, panic attacks, and all-encompassing rituals, these indicate an exacerbation requiring prompt attention.

Is Your Child Taking the Medication? If your child is not showing a positive response, then there are a number of things to consider. The first thing you need to think about is the medication. The initial step is to make sure that your child is taking the fully prescribed dosage. Double check the label to make sure you are following the instructions precisely. Make a chart where you can check off each

Make sure your child swallows every pill or drop of liquid medication.

dose as it's administered. With all you have to manage, it's easy to lose track. The chart will keep you focused. You must also carefully watch your child swallow every pill or spoonful of the medication. I learned this the hard way. Sammy had been steadily improving, and then he suddenly seemed to fall off a cliff. He continued to decompensate for several days before I discovered he had been hiding his pills under the couch cushions. Another thing to consider is whether your child might be cheeking his medication. "Cheeking the meds" is when a patient pushes the pill into his cheek with his tongue, then drinks the water to make it look as if the pill is being swallowed. Failing to take prescribed medication is one of the hallmarks of mental illness. Mental health patients routinely decide they do not need their medication any more, or come up with good excuses to avoid taking it. A major reason is because they feel badly about themselves. They see it as a flaw that they need pills to stay stable, so they hide or cheek their pills. If you run into snags like this, remind yourself that your sick child is doing the very best she can. Stay patient; you'll find your way back.

What the doctor says:

"Once liquid medicine expires, it can become as much as 60 percent less effective. In essence, the patient will be taking less and less active medicine every day."

David Band, MD

Is Your Child on the Right Medication? On the other hand, if you know that your child is taking all her medication and still there is no response, or if there are big regressions, there are a couple of things to consider. The first is that she is not on the correct antibiotic or has not been prescribed a high enough dose. Doctors who are not familiar with PANDAS often want to treat it with the dose ordinarily prescribed for the infection. This usually doesn't work. Ten days of penicillin may work for a typical strep infection, but this one isn't typical. The doctor needs to treat with large doses for an extended period of time. The second possibility is that your child is on the wrong psychotropic medication. As you will learn from reading the doctor interviews in the appendix, the antibiotic that consistently obtains the best response is extended release Augmentin. This is not information based on scientific studies

Consider whether your child needs a change in medication or dosage.

(none exist as of this writing), but rather based on clinical observations. If your child is not on Augmentin XR and is not allergic to penicillin (Augmentin is penicillin based), you might talk with your physician about making a change assuming the infection is strep. If your child is allergic to penicillin, then Azithromycin or Omnicef seem to be the antibiotics of choice. If your child is on psychotropic medication, perhaps it is not the right one for him. In particular, keep in mind that the SSRIs can exacerbate behaviors in certain children. Regardless of whether your child is on an SSRI or another psychotropic medication, a change may be needed.

What the doctor says:

"In prescribing Augmentin, I agree that there is a dose relation in terms of age, weight, and height. I just think it's higher. I will start with the lowest dose possible, but if I don't get a response within a week or two I will try a higher dose before I abandon treatment."

Catherine Nicolaides, MD

Has the Medication or Dosage Changed?

If your child's behavior has changed, can it be correlated with a change in medication or dosage? If you have either introduced a new medication or changed the dosage then that may account for the behaviors. Remember, psychotropic medications enter the brain. Even a slight change in a well-balanced mix may cause mood swings, anxiety, and an increased level of extreme behaviors.

FACT: Stopping the antibiotics cold turkey often accounts for behavioral exacerbations.

It's not always "PANDAS coming back." Issues regarding drug interactions and dosage should be one of the first things you consider. If the dosage of medication was increased or decreased shortly before the problematic behaviors appeared, you may need to return to the former dosage right away.

What About Another Infection? The next option to consider is whether your child might have contracted a different infection, which could be either bacterial or viral. Assuming you've tested for strep, have you considered mycoplasma or Lyme? Those have been known to cause behavioral symptoms. If he's been playing outside, perhaps he was bitten by a tick and contracted Lyme. If she is going to school on a regular basis, she may have picked up a bad cold, walking pneumonia, the flu, or mononucleosis. With a compromised immune system, your child may easily contract a secondary infection. It may not have been present at the outset, but it is there now. Treating one infection, but not the other may be the problem.

> **FACT:**
> *A PANDAS child gets behaviors as the symptom of an infection.*

For a PANDAS child, virtually any infection—bacterial or viral—can trigger a behavioral exacerbation. Remember, some children get a sore throat or fever. Your child gets behaviors as the symptoms of his infection.

What About Increased Exposure? Take a moment to consider whether your child has been in a situation that was more likely than others to expose him to infections that may trigger a backslide. As far as outside activities, you do not want your child to live in a bubble, but it's sensible to exercise an extra ounce of caution. Consider whether a particular situation is more likely to expose him to infections and whether there is something you might do to reduce the risk. If the grade school notifies you that there is a sudden strep outbreak, keep your child home for a few days. If your neighbor's child shows up for a sleepover coughing and wheezing, send her home. And if there has been a stomach virus going around, perhaps it might be best to pass on a friend's birthday party invitation. These may not be ideal solutions and missing a party is always a disappointment, but it's better than dealing with a behavioral exacerbation. And don't forget to monitor

What the doctor says:

"You can't imagine how many kids I've seen with flare-ups after they've been crawling around in ball pits at amusement parks."

Tanya Murphy, MD

the health of other family members. Your child's behavioral flare up may be a sign that someone else in the household is sick. Perhaps your child picked up a virus or bacteria from a family member who is asymptomatic.

What About Anxiety? Are there any emotional triggers that might be involved? When children are tired or under stress, behaviors often exacerbate. Could it be school related? If you've recently introduced school, perhaps it is too much for her. Maybe she can only handle a modified schedule. Are your child's teachers helpful and understanding, or do they think your child's behaviors are "bad choices?" Are there too many expectations being placed on your child from different sources? Does your child need a different educational plan as described in chapter 11, "Educational Impact?" Is the school team clear that the only goal at present is for your child to show up and have a decent day? Are your child's peers supportive of what he is going through, or do they call him names? Is there anything going on at home that might be causing anxiety?

How About Sleep? Is your child getting enough sleep? Has she taken on too many activities too quickly? Is she exhausted? Perhaps you need to cut back on her after-school activities. She needs rest to recover. Make sure the computer and television are shut down in the early evening to help create a calming environment that encourages rest.

Has Your Child's Diet Changed? At the outset, you will have implemented the dietary changes suggested in chapter 6, "Nutritional Considerations." Have your child's eating habits reverted? Perhaps you have let down your guard and become less vigilant. It's understandable. We all have a tendency to slack off a bit as things

What the doctor says:

"I find that if the parent returns the child to his previous diet, stops the supplements, in short fails to manage the condition on an ongoing basis, then PANDAS will return or perhaps another autoimmune dysfunction may develop.

Ali Carine, DO

improve and maybe some of the important changes have fallen by the wayside as your child was doing better. Is he eating sugar again? Have you reintroduced milk or gluten? Are you still using the juicer and blender to deliver nutrient-rich foods? And if you have not made these dietary changes yet, perhaps it's time to do so—right away.

What About Vaccines? One of the questions often asked is whether vaccines can trigger an exacerbation. There is no clear answer because there is no research on the topic of vaccines and PANDAS. However, many of the treating physicians, who support vaccinations in the general population, feel that vaccinations can aggravate the symptoms in PANDAS children by activating the immune factors and possibly causing the blood-brain barrier to become permeable. And it seems as if live vaccines may pose more of a risk. It's a risk benefit analysis because, for example, the flu itself may also create an exacerbation. For more discussions about vaccines, take a look at the individual opinions on vaccines that are offered by some of the doctors in the appendix.

Solving the Mysterious Backslide: Matt's Story

Matt had a classic case of PANDAS. As a fourth grader, he went to sleep one night as normal and woke up the next morning displaying obsessive behaviors and odd language patterns. He was consumed with accuracy, percentages, and time. Every answer he gave to a question was given precisely and multiple times. When his mom asked that morning, "What time did you wake up?" Matt answered, "Seven-oh-three, okay, okay, I'm lying, it was seven-oh-two, no seven-oh-four, okay I think it was seven-oh-three." At lunch when she asked, "How was your chocolate milk?" Matt answered, "Good, kinda good, a little good, okay it was good." At bedtime, Matt's mom said, "Time to brush your teeth and get ready for bed." Matt said, "I heard eighty percent of that, maybe eighty-five percent, no eighty percent, maybe ninety percent not eighty percent." These were the kinds of answers he gave to every simple question throughout the day.

Within forty-eight hours Matt's mom had called the pediatrician. Because Matt had only behaviors, no temperature or other physical symptoms to report, the scheduling nurse said she would need to set up a consult. Those were booking three weeks out. While they were waiting for the consult, Matt developed a fever. This bumped him up to a sick child visit, and they were seen immediately. A rapid throat swab came back positive for strep. Matt's pediatrician said he thought it was PANDAS, prescribed a Z-pack, and scheduled an after-hours consult for the next evening. At the consultation, he explained all about PANDAS and gave a ten-day prescription for amoxicillin to follow the Z-pack. He also ordered an MRI to make sure nothing was overlooked. Then he met with his staff to make sure that a case like this received appropriate attention in the future. The scheduling nurse apologized to Matt's mom and said it had been a good learning experience for everyone in the office.

FACT: *An MRI is a magnetic resonance imaging whereby internal body structures can be examined.*

Matt waited almost four months for the MRI because his case was not considered an emergency. When completed, it showed no indication of a brain tumor. The neurologist agreed that Matt probably had PANDAS. Matt was referred to a psychiatrist, who suggested starting with two amino acids to supplement the amoxicillin he was still taking. "But we might have to go to antidepressants if you don't see a response," he added. Matt's mom was reluctant to go that route without fully exploring antibiotic therapy. As the amoxicillin continued, Matt began to respond. After another month, Matt was back to baseline so antibiotics were discontinued. But one week later, the behaviors returned. After another three to four months on a prophylactic dose of amoxicillin, Matt was much improved. The antibiotics were discontinued again, and this time Matt maintained.

Matt's fifth-grade year was uneventful until February when the behaviors started to creep back. In March and April, he had a lot of anxiety, particularly related to separation. He would sometimes call his mom from the nurse's office to say he missed her, and to ask her to come have lunch with him. A throat culture for strep came back negative, so no antibiotics were prescribed. He finished the school year with difficulty. Over the summer, he had a low level of manageable behaviors and vomited a few times out of the blue.

During the first week of sixth grade, Matt's behaviors exploded. The exacerbation of verbal tics and obsessive behaviors was much more severe than in the past. Matt battled his way through the behaviors with the help of a psychologist. He suffered recurrent strep infections until December that were treated each time with amoxicillin. At that point, his tonsils were removed, but he continued to test positive for strep throughout the spring. In spite of treatment with amoxicillin, he continued to struggle behaviorally, and while he maintained academically, it was not his usual performance.

Matt's mom contacted me in May of Matt's sixth-grade year. She had read *Saving Sammy* and as a result she had persuaded the pediatrician to try Matt on long-term extended release Augmentin (Augmentin XR). We talked about the importance of having Matt take probiotics. She also wondered if I had heard whether generic Augmentin was as effective as the name brand. I told her a number of physicians had informed me there was no indication that the generic version of the medication was less effective, but parents reported the name brand was more effective.

Matt started at 1000mg of Augmentin XR per day. But it wasn't until the second week, when the dose increased to 2000mg that Matt began to respond. His tics and obsessions faded away. Remaining on that dose of Augmentin XR until December, Matt had eight solid months of recovery. His teachers remarked on how positive his seventh-grade academic performance was from the prior year. Then, in late December, he had what the family felt was a minor cold with a runny nose and coughing. During January, his stress level rose. Tests, projects, and school sports participation all produced anxiety. The family knew things were generally more stressful in seventh grade, but then he said he was feeling, "the way I used to." By the end of January he was having emotional breakdowns. Matt was back at the pediatrician's. His rapid strep test was positive, and his mom reached out to me again.

Having lived the wave of Sammy's recovery, I fully understood when Matt's mom was beside herself with grief. It's always scary when you think you have this horrible disorder managed, and it rears its ugly head again. We talked over all the different possibilities that might have triggered the exacerbation. She mentioned that there was strep in the school. I explained that for a child like Matt, even when on antibiotics, the mere presence of strep in others might trigger his immune system. "It's almost like a peanut allergy," I explained. "They just can't be around it." I pointed out that Sammy had never attended school during the year of his recovery, which gave his immune system a complete rest from the typical infections spread by middle schoolers from one to another. Matt's mom said he was taking 2000mg Augmentin XR per day. He was having no bowel issues handling that dose, so the pediatrician was considering adding a third pill of either 500mg or perhaps 1000mg.

Matt was stressing over his performance on the school basketball team. We talked about having a conversation with him about how important it was to let go of that anxiety. Placing additional stressors on an overtaxed immune system would not help him. I also suggested that she be sure to compliment him on the insight he had shown by recognizing the infection was probably back. They had most likely intervened early enough that the behaviors would not reach the heightened level they had reached eight months earlier. I was suspicious of the December "cold" though. It might have been just that, or it might have been a precursor of the infection returning. More important, I wondered if it might have been an indication of something else; perhaps mycoplasma, the bacteria involved in walking pneumonia. Matt had been diagnosed on the basis of throat swabs. I mentioned that if Matt were my son, I'd want blood work for ASO and Anti-DNase B titers so that I'd have a measure for future comparisons. And if they did blood work, I'd also want blood tests for mycoplasma pneumonia (IgG and IgM titers).

We also discussed inflammation, the blood-brain barrier, and nutrition. I gave her a thumbnail sketch of the foods to watch out for, first and foremost sugar. "Matt really likes his sugar," she said. "He eats a good, healthy meal, but he always wants dessert. Sometimes he'll have two a day." We agreed those desserts needed to stop. I also suggested that she take a look at what Matt might be drinking during his basketball games because many of those "power" drinks are laden with sugar.

Two weeks later, Matt's mom faxed me copies of Matt's blood work. Matt's strep titers were normal, but the mycoplasma was elevated. "The school nurse told me today there was a recent case of mycoplasma," she said tearfully. I recommended that she take Matt to see the pediatrician right away because once the immune system establishes certain pathways to the brain, it seems that any infection—bacterial or viral—can cause the behaviors to return. And mycoplasma will not respond to a penicillin-based antibiotic such as Augmentin.

With the appropriate treatment for both strep and mycoplasma in place, Matt was improving within a week or two. More than a year later, he continues to do well. Matt and his mom remain alert to look out for the first sign of a problem. They both know that his symptoms of an infection are behavioral. If those behaviors rear their ugly heads, they know it means he needs antibiotics. Most important, Matt knows that he can bring this to his mother, and she will make sure he receives the appropriate treatment.

SUMMING IT UP

Children recover at their own pace and often have a few backslides along the way. When that happens it's frightening, but with patience you can probably figure out what's causing the exacerbation. Sit down with a pen and paper, review all the questions listed above, and write down the answers based on your child's situation. Chances are you will find the answer. Then call your PANDAS doctor to consult by telephone or meet to figure out what the next step will be. You will get through this, and sometimes the answer is as simple as running another blood test to look for a different infection.

Nonetheless, if you have eliminated all of the above as possibilities, then you may have to discuss more invasive measures with your doctor. If you have given high-dose, long-term antibiotics a full and fair chance to address the disorder, and you have implemented the recommended dietary changes, then you may need to consider IV Ig or plasmapheresis if your child is not responding as you had hoped. These procedures are usually ordered by doctors with a specialty in particular areas of medicine, usually neurology, immunology, or allergy. IV Ig and plasmapheresis are more fully described in chapter 4, "Medical Treatment."

BIG IDEAS FROM CHAPTER TEN

❑ Recovery comes in waves, and you must stay positive throughout the ups and downs.

❑ The time it takes to reach full recovery will depend on how early PANDAS was recognized.

❑ There is a difference between a temporary backslide and having your child lose all of her hard-won gains.

❑ You must intervene with medical attention if your child is consistently losing her gains.

❑ Consider whether there are any changes in these four key areas of the child's life that may be contributing to the behavioral problems:

medical
emotional
nutritional
exposure to infections.

Educational Impact

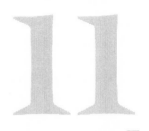

Dear Beth,

I know you're a lawyer. Do you ever work with parents who need help with their school systems? Our little boy is so sick with PANDAS that he cannot leave the house. The school system wants us to force him into the car, drive him to school, have school personnel carry him into the school building, and then restrain him until the fight-flight response subsides. Have you ever heard of such a thing? Can they make us do that? All we want is home tutoring for our son until he is well.

Outraged!

Dear Outraged,

The school system cannot force you to do that and, in my opinion, what they are suggesting may amount to child abuse. If your son is unable to leave your home, then the school system has to provide tutoring and, yes, I can help you.

Beth

There is a time for children to go to school, and there is a time when they need to stay home. If your child is desperately ill, can't make it out the front door, has stopped eating, won't bathe or change his clothes, and is otherwise struggling on a daily basis, then school may not be the best place for him. This may be contrary to the professional advice you are receiving, but I am speaking from personal experience. Before Sammy was correctly diagnosed with PANDAS, I was consistently advised that it was important for him to keep going to school. Although my heart never believed it was the right thing for him, I tried. I kept taking him back and forth, assuming the professionals knew what was best. Most days, when we finally arrived, he couldn't even make it out of the van. Eventually, even our Herculean attempts proved impossible. We gave up. He felt like a failure. I felt defeated. Broken hearts were all we had to show for our efforts.

Your child is not going to stay away from school forever, but it may be what he needs now. Alternatively, he may not be able to be there everyday or he may need special accommodations while he is there in order to be successful. This chapter outlines the educational considerations and rights that apply to PANDAS children. By reading it, you will become a more effective educational advocate for your child.

Is School the Best Place?

PANDAS seems as if your child has been in a major accident, but you can't find the truck that hit him. It's a good analogy to keep in mind. Because if your child had been in a massive accident, we wouldn't expect to see him back in school anytime soon. And that's what PANDAS feels like to a child; as if he's been slammed by an invisible truck. Even if we could get that accident victim to school, would we really want him there? What about the risk of getting his broken bones bumped, his bruised head banged, and his aching torso jostled in the ordinary tug and pull of a routine school day? There's a similar risk of injury for PANDAS children, but it isn't so easy to see. It's the risk of contracting another infection and further taxing the immune system.

The decision of whether your child needs to stay home is one carefully made after weighing the risks and the benefits of being in school. First you must gauge the severity of the illness. Is your child well enough to function in a school setting right now? Of course she is not going to stay home forever. Yes, she might "pick something up" even at the doctor's office, and it's also possible that her sibling might bring home the flu and infect the entire family. But can your child engage in what the school has to offer and is the risk of school a wise one to take right now? Maybe your child is not physically healthy enough to navigate her way through that giant petri dish of bacteria and viruses called school. Think of the number of children who are sent to school sick, full of germs to spread, because both parents are working to make ends meet and there's no one to stay home and care for a sick child. It's quite possible that—for now—school simply may not be a safe place for your child. Maybe your PANDAS child's immune system needs to rest and rebuild. Sammy was so debilitated that he stayed home for two full years. Perhaps that's part of why he fully recovered. He struggled to beat the disorder and overcome the behaviors, but he did not have to struggle against other infections.

You must also consider the emotional impact. What is the social environment at your child's school? Is there a psychological risk of potentially being subjected to ridicule from unkind peers? Will your

FACT:

If your child is not well enough to attend school right now, try to keep her connected with her favorite peers and activities. These will be her motivations to return.

school step in to stop any bullying, or will your child be facing another challenge to overcome? You need to decide what is right for your child, but—honestly—in the greater scheme of life, missing school for a while is not a catastrophe. And if your child is too sick to meaningfully participate, what's the point of being there?

If your child does need to be home for a while, remember that it's temporary. Once it's feasible, pencil in a projected return date. The date may need to shift, but having a date gives everyone involved a target to work toward. If the date seems unlikely as it approaches, push it back. It is not carved in stone and adjusting the target is not a failure; it's smart. Just keep in mind that the longer a child is out of school, the more difficult and awkward it will be to eventually return, so never lose sight of that goal. During the homebound period, take advantage of any opportunities that may be available to keep your child engaged with peers. A PANDAS child needs motivation, something that he or she wants to return to: friends, clubs, gymnastics, chorus, school plays, art exhibits, class projects, sports, recitals. Help your child stay connected to the parts of life that cause him to thrive. Giving him reasons to want to rejoin his classmates will motivate him and make his re-entry easier.

Now let's get started on the nuts and bolts of what you need to know to work well with your child's school during this difficult time.

What to Say

1. Share the Information. Your child is entitled to an education whether she is physically at school or at home due to illness. Working effectively with your child's school is important to achieving this goal. PANDAS is nothing to be ashamed of and should not be a secret. Parents are not embarrassed if their child has cancer or diabetes, and you should not be embarrassed about PANDAS. Your child has an immune dysfunction that you are working on healing, and it presents itself as a behavioral disorder. Teachers need to know what is going on. They spend a great deal of time with your child. They are well educated and usually caring. Give them the information they need to help your child succeed.

Because PANDAS can be complicated, keep your initial explanation simple: "My child has a common infection that, in some children, causes behaviors. It's basically rheumatic fever of the brain, and his behaviors are the symptoms of the disorder. The acronym for what he has is PANDAS. Fortunately, he'll get better but it may take a while." From there, you can offer more detailed explanations, but keep coming back to the simplest denominator: your child's brain is under assault and that causes the behaviors the teacher will see. Give the teacher examples of those behaviors. Explain that you are working with your child's doctor to manage this disorder, but you need the teacher's help because the information he or she can provide is invaluable.

2. Ask the Teacher for Help. The degree of your child's illness will determine how involved the school will become in helping you. If it's mild and the behaviors are manageable, you may simply need to maintain a good relationship with the classroom teacher. Set up a separate time to meet with the teacher, explain briefly about PANDAS, and describe how it manifests behaviorally in your child. Ask to be notified if there is a strep outbreak, or if many kids are suddenly out sick for other reasons. Also ask to be apprised if the teacher notices any behaviors returning: obsessions, tics, anxiety, changes in handwriting, a decline in math skills, and so forth. This will help you determine whether medical interventions may be needed. You will also need to inform others at school who may be keys to helping with recovery, particularly the school nurse.

3. Inform the School Nurse. School nurses are often advocates for PANDAS and may become one of your child's strongest allies. They understand autoimmune diseases and, if not already familiar with PANDAS, will understand when you explain that PANDAS is rheumatic fever of the brain. The nurse's office may also provide refuge. Some children simply need a place that feels safe to carry out a compulsion or tic that they've been holding in check during class. Your child may not feel comfortable visiting a school counselor or social worker during a behavioral exacerbation, but a nurse who understands the medical condition may be a more comfortable option. School nurses do an excellent job tracking visits, which will be important information to share with your child's doctor. Are the child's visits to the nurse increasing, a possible sign that anxiety and compulsions are rising? Or are the visits decreasing, thus indicating that treatment is working? How long is a typical visit to the nurse's office for your child? What does your child tell the nurse and what time of the school day does he or she most often visit? By studying the data, you may be able to find patterns and pinpoint which part of the day is most difficult. This information may lead you to figure out why.

> **FACT:**
> *The school nurse may be one of your child's strongest allies.*

4. Talk with the School Counselor. Your child is probably working with a Cognitive Behavioral Therapist and may not want to talk with school personnel about PANDAS. But keeping the school-based counselor informed is wise because your child may need a place to go from time to time to regroup. If your child does want to talk, an informed counselor can at least offer comfort during the tough times. The counselor may also be a resource for your other children. Siblings need to be able to share with someone outside the home about what they are going through. Find out what the school has to offer for them. Grade schools often have groups for youngsters to discuss divorce, friendship, and other potentially difficult issues. Sometimes they have lunch with the school counselor once a week. There might be a group that would work well for your grade schooler, or perhaps the counselor might be available to just talk. Middle and high school social workers, counselors, and peer support groups can be a source of support at that age level. If the school knows what is going on in the home, they will have a better understanding if your other children start to show signs of having their own difficult time.

5. Approaching Others. With the school nurse and counselor in your corner, you'll be in a good position to meet with others. As you speak with them, some may find it difficult to accept that an infection can cause mental illness. When doubt is cast, I mention syphilis because it is well known that untreated syphilis causes serious mental health issues. For those who want more information about the disorder, recommend the websites of the NIMH and the International OCD Foundation. Suggest they read *Saving Sammy*.

> *Dear Beth,*
>
> *I wanted to share some of the things that have helped me keep track of what is going on with my son at school. I have asked the school to keep me apprised by e-mail once a week about his behaviors. I let them know what I am seeing at home and ask if they are seeing it at school. I try to be specific: "This week I am seeing an increase in tics at home. Have you noticed anything?" Then I print the responses and bring them to doctor appointments. This record helps me in getting the pediatrician and his other doctors to listen more carefully. I also schedule informal meetings with his team or sometimes just to sit with the teachers. I think that showing up in person makes the schools take it a little more seriously and helps get them to stay on top of sending me e-mails to print. Teachers can get so burnt out, and the last thing they want is a child who is having uncontrolled behaviors in their classroom. I learned that taking the really nice, "I am working with the pediatrician and want to do everything I can to help my child along with his school environment," approach really helps. And being an active parent in my son's education helps me collect the data that I need. My son also has a case manager because of his ADHD and autism. Mine keeps very detailed notes, and I call her when PANDAS symptoms are flaring up. Case managers will go to doctor appointments and can write up timelines etc. I feel the more outside professionals that can write about the child's symptoms, the more likely a doctor is going to listen. The more papers documenting symptoms from people other than parents the better (I think). I hope this helps.*
>
> *Successful School Mom*

Establishing an Educational Program

It will always prove fruitful to have positive relations with the school-based professionals involved in your children's lives. As is true with doctors, you want to be the parent they want most to help. If you have years of a solid relationship with your children's teachers and the administration, they already know that the information you bring them is reliable. If you do not have that history in place when your child becomes ill, then you will need to build a relationship. It may not be easy, but it's part of your job. You always have the option to change doctors, but moving to a new school system is often impossible. Your PANDAS child may need a modified school schedule, additional support, home-based tutoring, help with work, quiet time to regroup, and a host of other accommodations to help during his period of recovery. If so, you will need a comprehensive plan to meet your child's needs. Your child is entitled to a free appropriate public education and part of your responsibility is to make sure he gets it. You can threaten your school system with lawsuits and bring in advocates; but at the end of the day what you need is help, not another battle. If you can avoid one, that will be ideal.

FACT: Having a strong, positive relationship with your school system will help you get what you need for your child.

In Sammy's situation, we had all the right ingredients. I had years of history with the school system, a solid foundation with the administrators, and people who wanted to do what they could to help. We were blessed. I know that not all of you are so fortunate. Some school systems are extremely difficult and stern measures are needed to get things properly on track for children in need of educational services. Understanding the basic parameters of education law will help you figure out whether you can work with your school system or whether you will need to bring in someone to help.

The rest of this chapter describes the two federal laws that may be instrumental in helping to get your child the education he needs:

Individuals with Disabilities Education Improvement Act of 2004

Section 504 of the Rehabilitation Act of 1973

The Way It Should Be

When Sammy was sick, our school system worked hard to try to develop a plan that would work. Eventually, when it was clear that attending school was not an option, he received home-based tutoring. Susan Martin was the director of special services for our school system at the time. She remains in that position for the Maine Regional School Unit 21 serving Arundel-Kennebunk-Kennebunkport with 2,640 students. Even before Sammy was ill, I knew her to be professional and thorough. For help writing about the viewpoint of a school system, I turned to Ms. Martin.

Ms. Martin began her career in special education in 1981, first as a teacher and then as a special education administrator in 1994. She agreed to allow me to weave her knowledge and perspective on educational rights throughout this section. I approached her because she was so supportive about making sure that Sammy got what he needed. I know that you are not all so fortunate as to have someone like Ms. Martin on your team, but perhaps reviewing this information and the insight she offers will model what you need.

Ms. Martin's enthusiasm for her position and devotion to the children she serves is inspiring. "We try to create an individual program for each student and have really good staff who are willing to be creative people," Ms. Martin said. "When a child with a unique profile comes into the district, we pull resources from all the schools. We try to put together a team that will support the child, because we really want the child to succeed. We're not trying to push children into programs. We're trying to create ones that work for them. I always find it interesting because every child's different, so it's a challenge, a new project every time."

Legal Considerations

There are two areas of federal law that may apply to PANDAS children: the Individuals with Disabilities Education Improvement Act of 2004 (IDEA) and Section 504 of the Rehabilitation Act of 1973. Each law provides unique protections, and they are summarized in the sections below. Generally, the IDEA provides for individualized instruction for children who have special needs. The services cover

Section 504 may be the quickest path to getting educational help for your child.

all educational areas; for example a child may require special education services for reading or mathematics. Qualifying under the IDEA for special services can be a lengthy process given the required testings, evaluations, and eligibility determinations that are required. Section 504 qualification is less formal and moves more quickly. Under Section 504, each student is entitled to equal access to an education and adjustments need to be made if there are conditions that interfere with equal access. For example, Section 504 would apply to a child with ADHD who needs help keeping track of assignments through a notebook that travels between home and school. Section 504 may offer an alternative route to obtain prompt help while testing is pursued for IDEA qualification.

FACT:
Public schools are required to comply with the IDEA and Section 504 because these are federal laws and the schools receive federal funds. Private schools do not receive federal funds so there is no similar obligation.

Each state enacts regulations to ensure that its school systems comply with these federal laws. The educational obligations apply to public schools because they receive federal funds. Private schools have no similar legal obligations. There are some private schools that are quite good about addressing the needs of a PANDAS child, but there are others that may ask you to withdraw your child simply because they are not set up to address atypical needs. Public school systems have teachers specially trained in delivering special services, typically private schools do not. For example, there is no legal obligation imposed on private schools to furnish their students with home-based tutoring should the student's illness warrant that service.

Individuals with Disabilities Education Improvement Act of 2004 (IDEA). Under the IDEA, schools must ensure that children with disabilities are provided a free appropriate public education (FAPE) in the least restrictive educational environment possible. Children who receive services under IDEA are commonly known to be receiving "special education." Children who are identified as having learning or physical disabilities are referred to an individualized education program team (IEP team); then they are referred for professional evaluations. The results of the evaluations will be reviewed and discussed at a meeting of the IEP team. Parents are members of the team. Determinations for eligibility are made at the

FACT: *Children with disabilities are entitled to receive special education under the IDEA.*

meeting. Considering the determinations, the team then writes an individualized education program (an IEP) for the child. This will specify the individualized special instruction the child will receive. For example, a child with a learning disability in reading might be given a different reading program from the rest of the class and one-on-one time with a skilled tutor. Parents must be included in all stages of this process and have the right to request mediation, file a complaint, or request a due process hearing if they do not agree with the various outcomes. The IEP is reviewed on a periodic basis and adjusted as needed.

The IDEA and related requirements will apply to your PANDAS child if she has an IEP in place when she becomes sick. For example, if she has a disability in reading and individualized instruction is being provided pursuant to an IEP, the provisions of the IEP will continue to apply. It may be tougher for your child to qualify for special education if no issues were identified prior to the onset of PANDAS. It may only be in retrospect that you recognize the significance of, for example, the fine motor deterioration and quirky stuff with math and spelling that were earlier chalked up to "odd." Don't discount the possibility of being able to achieve special education for your child, but in the meantime Section 504 should definitely apply.

Section 504 of the Rehabilitation Act of 1973 (Section 504).
What about a child who does not have an IEP when PANDAS strikes? "I would think that any district at some level will have to help under Section 504," said Ms. Martin, "because if a child with a physical or mental impairment that substantially limits a major life activity is not able to access his education then accommodations *have* to be made. That's law, too, maybe even stronger law than IDEA."

Section 504 is quite broad. Any child with an IEP automatically has the protections of Section 504, but a child who becomes "disabled" can qualify for Section 504 protections even if he does not need specialized instruction. In other words, the hypothetical child who was in a bad accident and cannot come to school for an extended period of time will qualify under Section 504, even if he's the brightest kid in his class. The plan developed to address needs under Section 504 is called a "504 Plan." It covers the adjustments or "accommodations" that will be made to help your child succeed.

Section 504 provides equal access for education and covers a wide range of needs—from those that are either relatively straightforward to those more complicated. "I've always used the term 'to bring it to a level playing field' for 504," said Ms. Martin, "because that's what it's about." A child with ADHD may have a 504 Plan with preferential seating or a requirement that someone help with organizing notes. A child with a debilitating illness who cannot come to school will have a 504 Plan that calls for homebound instruction. Children with seizure disorders, severe asthma, and serious depression are all protected by Section 504. Some plans are very extensive and detailed, covering what must happen in certain circumstances, who needs to be trained, and the steps to follow if the child is, for example, on a field trip when an issue presents itself. But the plans tend to be, "far simpler," than an IEP according to Ms. Martin because, "it's more the school will do this, the student will do that, and the parent will do this, so it's not as lengthy. But it is an agreement of what we are going to do so that this kiddo can access his education." The changes that are made to enable that access are called "accommodations."

Section 504 covers a student who has a physical or mental impairment that substantially limits one or more major life activities and is generally expected to last for a period of time. If you carefully read the definition, you will see that a PANDAS child qualifies. A "mental impairment" is any mental or psychological disorder. A "major life activity" includes "the operation of a major bodily function." "Function of the immune system" is recognized as "the operation of a major bodily function," as are the brain and neurological functions. Reference is made to the *DSM* for identification of the mental impairment, but that is not a requirement. And although PANDAS is not in the *DSM* the symptoms of PANDAS—obsessions, compulsions, ADHD, anxiety, depression and

> **FACT:**
> *A PANDAS child qualifies for accommodations under Section 504.*

so forth—certainly are. Given the immune system dysfunction and the psychological symptoms of your PANDAS child, and assuming she is having difficulty accessing her education, she should meet the requirements for a 504 Plan. The Plan will cover the accommodations that will be made to your child's educational program.

As a parent, you are able to initiate a request for a 504 Plan. You should contact your school district to find out its procedures for doing so. Ultimately, the process will be similar to that which results in an IEP, but without the need for extensive evaluations. A meeting will be convened to review the circumstances. You will be invited to attend. If you don't agree with the decisions, your rights to object are similar to those under the IDEA.

Educational Meetings

The key to success at any meeting is preparation. The more you understand your rights, the limitations on those rights, and what you want to achieve at the meeting, the more successful you will be. One mistake that I find parents make is to think that when a parent presents the problem, the school system will have the solution. Sometimes this is true, but more often the school will be looking to you to make suggestions. If your child is the hypothetical one hit by a truck who can't leave the house, the school will know it has to provide homebound instruction. But chances are that PANDAS is new to the school. You need to be the one person in the room who has the information and is crystal clear.

Whether your school meeting is being held for an IEP or a 504 Plan, it's possible that such meetings may be intimidating at first. The clarity of knowing your rights and your goals will help you feel more comfortable. You should expect that there may be up to

You are the person who knows your child best, so bring suggestions to the meeting of what accommodations will help your child to do better. Bringing along ideas will also demonstrate how much you care and want to work with others.

eight professionals in the room, including the special services director, classroom teachers, special education teachers, school psychologist, school social worker, and others. Keep in mind that they have all been to many of these meetings. Sometimes it seems that they are speaking a different language. It's okay to ask questions about anything you do not understand, and you should take notes if that makes it easier. Asking questions and taking notes shows how much you care about your child. You may even want to record the meeting if you think it would be helpful to listen to everything again. Remember: how you conduct yourself at these meetings is just as important as how you conduct yourself with your child's doctors.

You can also bring along others who have knowledge about your child. While it's unlikely you'll be able to persuade your child's physician or psychologist to attend (unless by speakerphone), you should ask them to please provide you with a diagnosis in writing that will help you with the meetings. Some will make specific recommendations such as attending school on a modified schedule. Submit these written recommendations in advance and keep a copy for yourself.

School meetings are designed for gathering information, sharing it with everyone present, and making team decisions about how best to move forward. You need to carefully think through in advance what you hope to gain from the meeting and attend with suggestions of specific changes that you believe might help your child. Keep three things in mind when you attend a school meeting. First, this is your child and she is your responsibility. Second, what's happened is not the school's fault. Third, although those with special education training have studied disorders and the theories of how best to address them, few have lived with a child as ill as yours. You may need to educate the team about what life is like on a daily basis with a PANDAS child.

Unfortunately, if the goal of the school system is to deny providing services—and that is the approach of some—the environment at these meetings can feel hostile. If you anticipate that type of situation, you may want to arrange for an educational advocate or an attorney to attend with you and have that person do the follow up.

There is no blanket set of accommodations that will apply for all PANDAS children. You know your child best and need to consider in advance what may help. Make a list, bring it with you, and advocate for those accommodations. The questions you may want to consider are:

- ❑ What will make your child's daily life easier?
- ❑ Is attending a full day of school every day so difficult that he needs a modified schedule?
- ❑ Does he need a quiet place to go and collect himself when his anxiety becomes overwhelming?
- ❑ Does he need periodic breaks throughout the day?
- ❑ Is homework so difficult that he needs a waiver?
- ❑ Does he need tutoring?
- ❑ Are his classmates understanding or bullying?

The web is a good source for developing the list of accommodations that may be helpful for your child. If you search by your child's diagnosis or main disability (i.e. accommodations for ADD) you will be able to find helpful suggestions. At this point the list is short when you search accommodations for PANDAS. But remember that it is the symptoms of PANDAS you are trying to address: distractibility, tics, OCD. If you search for accommodations specifically to address those symptoms, you will find a wealth of information. Also, don't waste time or confuse an accommodation with what is just plain good teaching. Good teaching should be expected, not listed as an accommodation. "Positive reinforcement" is frequently used as an accommodation, but we should expect that on a daily basis. Clearly state the difference in teaching that your child needs as opposed to the skills that are part of good teaching. "Multi-modal presentation" is a catchphrase that often shows up in 504 Plans and is simply part of good teaching. Instead, state clearly what works best for your child: "visual models of the finished product" or "visual models paired with verbal directions."

Once you have your draft list compiled, your next step is to prioritize. Which accommodations will make the most difference in your child's life? Depending on your child's age, you may want to sit down and review them together. Be prepared to push for what really matters. Let the others go.

> *Dear Beth,*
> *You might also want to mention to parents that "less is more."*
> *Parents want the most relevant, important accommodations to be*
> *highlighted. It can be tempting to go overboard on a lengthy list of*
> *accommodations, especially if they seem like great solutions. However,*
> *the IEP or 504 Plan then becomes a bunch of words and not a usable,*
> *working document. Parents want classroom teachers to read it and*
> *actively implement the accommodations, keeping the most relevant*
> *and effective in their minds.*
> *I know it from all sides because my son has PANDAS, he needed*
> *accommodations, and I am a special education teacher.*
> *Special Teaching Mom*

SUMMING IT UP

By having read this chapter, you should be able to identify the pros and cons of having your child attend school at present, be familiar with your child's legal right to be educated, and understand how to effectively participate in getting your child what he or she needs to succeed educationally. You are the best person to identify your child's specific needs, and it may be the solutions that work best will be those you bring to the team meeting. When you meet, be aware that the finances and resources of school systems are always stretched. The more you can offer practical solutions with minimal cost, the more receptive you may find the team. Nonetheless, if your child simply cannot leave the house then home-based tutoring will be the only solution.

There are three equal ingredients in addressing your child's needs; the tone set by the person in charge of your school system's special services, the resources the school system has at its disposal, and you. Ms. Martin eloquently described this when she said, "As with any business meeting or partnership you go into, it depends how the parties approach the table. There are directors who approach the process in a negative sense of, 'You're not getting one cent out of us.' But while you always have to be fiscally responsible, you have to remember you're there for the kids. And you're charged by the law with creating the most appropriate program that you can."

In summary, be thoroughly prepared. However, if you have no success in getting what your child needs from your school system in spite of your best efforts, you may need to think about hiring an attorney.

BIG IDEAS FROM CHAPTER ELEVEN

❏ School may not be the best place for your PANDAS child when he is very sick.
❏ Sharing information with the school is important to your child's recovery.
❏ Even children who cannot attend school are entitled to a free appropriate public education.
❏ If your child is well enough to physically attend, the school may still need to make special accommodations so that your child can successfully receive an education.
❏ There are two areas of the law that may apply to the education of a PANDAS child:
    Individuals with Disabilities Education Improvement Act of 2004 (IDEA)
    Section 504 of the Rehabilitation Act of 1973.
❏ IDEA covers students who need special help with academics.
❏ An IEP describes the special services the child receives under IDEA.
❏ Section 504 covers students who are unable to access their education without help.
❏ A 504 Plan describes the accommodations that will be made to help the child.
❏ Generally, if a child does not already have an IEP in place when he gets sick, he will probably not receive special services as a result of developing PANDAS, but he will be covered under Section 504.
❏ For both IDEA and Section 504, the parent or primary caregiver may initiate the process.

V BUMPS ALONG THE WAY

Supports and Conflict

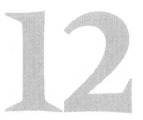

Dear Beth,

My son is so sick with compulsions that he can't leave the house. The only time he ever got better was when he was on antibiotics for strep throat. I think it's PANDAS, but the doctors say there's no connection. My husband wants me to stop talking about PANDAS. My other children think my son is faking it. Family members think I'm a bad mother, and the teachers think I don't want him in school. I don't know what to do or where to turn. I know you must hear from so many parents, but if you could write back it would mean so much to me. I feel so alone.

Helpless

Dear Helpless,

You are not alone. There are many parents facing the same issues as you. Have you thought of joining a support group? Groups are meeting nationwide, and you can find one by visiting the pull down menu of Other Resources on savingsammy.net

Beth

Feeling alone is such a tough place to be, especially when what you need most is emotional support. It is often a struggle to maintain positive, nurturing relationships with your partner, other children, extended family members, and friends when caring for a sick child. It's even more discouraging when there is conflict over appropriate medical care. This chapter discusses the strain that PANDAS places on relationships and offers direction about how you can build the support network you need during this difficult time.

Finding Support

> **FACT:**
> *The medical community is not always right. There have been major mistakes made in medicine that have lasted for many years and cost many patients their lives. Two examples are childbed fever and stomach ulcers.*

Research shows that most health-care decisions in the United States are made by women, so it makes sense that moms usually take the lead in seeking treatment for their PANDAS children. Dads sometimes take on this role and more are stepping up every day, but mostly it is moms who handle their child's health-care needs. What makes PANDAS much tougher than other illnesses is the controversy that surrounds it. As difficult as it may be to manage juvenile diabetes, no one will tell you it doesn't exist. When parents— married, never married, divorced, or step-parenting—have a difference of opinion over treatment and diagnosis, coupled with the conflicting opinions of different doctors, the situation becomes full of friction on both fronts: home and medical. A healthy dose of each approach is helpful, but when parents squabble over their divergent positions it is the child who suffers. Even when the parents are united, they may find themselves at odds with other family members.

If you are facing this challenge, remind yourself and others that doctors are not always right. The medical community has historically made some very big mistakes in medicine that have cost many lives. Knowing a few examples may help you feel comfortable with the fact that the doctors who adamantly claim PANDAS doesn't exist are not correct.

One big mistake in medicine that killed many women was the resistance to the true cause of "childbed fever." During the 1800s, women were dying in droves after delivering babies in hospitals. Why? The reason was because doctors refused to wash between patients and procedures. They often performed autopsies and then went from bed to bed examining pregnant women and delivering babies. An apron splattered with blood and pus was considered a sign of status. During the 1840s, two distinguished physicians independently proposed that women were dying because doctors were spreading infections. Dr. Oliver Wendell Holmes in the United

States and Dr. Igzna Semmelweis in Austria both wanted doctors to wash their hands and change clothing between patients. They were both ridiculed. "Doctors are gentlemen," said Dr. Charles Meigs of the Jefferson College of Medicine in Philadelphia, "and gentlemen's hands are clean." Dr. Semmelweis reported that childbed fever deaths were reduced by 90 percent when doctors simply washed with an antiseptic solution before deliveries. His data was deemed insufficient scientific proof by the greater medical community, so women continued to die into the 1900s. And what was the bacteria spread by the doctors and causing death? It was group A strep.

A more recent big mistake was stomach ulcers. It took twenty years for the medical community to accept the fact that peptic stomach ulcers are caused by bacteria. The medical community's position was that bacteria could not survive in the stomach. Patients continued to suffer and die until Australian physician Dr. Barry Marshall infected himself with the bacteria H-pylori, developed the ulcers, cured himself with antibiotics, and thus demonstrated that it was a bacterial infection causing the ulcers. He and his medical partner won the Nobel Prize in Medicine in 2005.

You know from reading this book and probably from your own research that there is plenty of evidence-based medicine to support PANDAS. Don't let an obstinate practitioner or uneducated naysayer cause you to question your course. Remind those who challenge you that up to 35 percent of mothers died following childbirth while they were waiting for medical doctors to agree that washing their hands between deliveries could save lives.

Your child does not have time to wait.

The Discipline Dispute

Dear Beth,

My son has had fifteen strep infections in the past two years. His OCD and tics are so bad that it's hard for him to walk. The doctors say there's no such thing as PANDAS and will only put him on antibiotics for ten days if his throat test is positive. I finally got them to run a blood test and the titer is over 800, but they said it's a coincidence. My husband and the rest of our family say it's my fault for not being strict enough when he was little. Could that really be it?

So Sad

> *Dear Sad,*
> *Your child has indisputable evidence of a serious infection. Your parenting skills are not the reason why your little guy is sick. Find different doctors and don't listen to that nonsense.*
> *Beth*

FACT:
Blame, family conflict, and lack of cohesion in the home are all stumbling blocks to recovery.

When a parent is confronted by an unsupportive family member, a frequent focus is discipline. Parents are told (by each other, by family members, by professionals) that if parental discipline had been sufficient when the child was little, he'd be just fine now. "Send him to me for a week, and I'll straighten him out," is a favorite refrain. Then there are relentless, hurtful comparisons to other family members and even neighbors with scores of sunny-faced children who are excelling at school and developing Olympic-contender athletic abilities. While the parent keeps plowing ahead, trying to figure out if there's an infection-based reason for the child's behaviors, he or she is told it's excuses being sought for earlier deficient parenting skills.

Eventually, as a result of financial constraints, emotional abuse, resulting debilitation, and uncaring doctors, some parents give up and the child stays sick. That's not your story, though, because you are either in a supportive relationship with your child's other parent or you are going to find the supports and strength you need to press forward. Keep in mind that legally, unless there is a court order to the contrary, either parent has the right to seek medical treatment for the child. Furthermore, neither parent has the right to exercise his or her individual rights in such a way that it keeps the child ill.

There are some truly horrendous situations. More than one PANDAS child's mother has been accused of Munchausen's by Proxy. Munchausen's by Proxy (MBP) is when a parent, most often a mother, fakes an illness in her child. The MBP mother takes the child from doctor to doctor until she manages to convince someone that the child is ill with whatever symptoms the parent has concocted. If you find yourself facing this type of accusation, understand that there is an important distinction between you and a Munchausen parent: there is no disagreement about the fact that your child is sick, the only question is why. PANDAS parents firmly believe their children can get well, but that they are not getting the right treatment.

If you are in a relationship with an unsupportive partner or other family member, here are some suggestions you might consider. These are geared more toward survival than relationship building. I'm not a trained therapist and there is certainly a professional who may be able to provide better help, but it's doubtful you

You may need to stop seeking support from family members and look elsewhere for assistance and understanding.

have time to sit with a therapist and sort this out. Perhaps one of these steps may help you keep going until the situation resolves itself one way or the other.

1. Join a Support Group. There are PANDAS support groups meeting across the country. The meetings are filled with plenty of parents who are willing to share their stories and offer you their connections. Don't be shy. Support group members have lived your journey and will offer you tremendous help and comfort. Learn from them. If you visit savingsammy.net you will find a list of these groups. If you cannot find a local support group, search the web for resources. There are multiple websites and Facebook pages all devoted to PANDAS, which may be of help to you. Many are listed at the back of this book under "Additional Resources."

2. Stop Defending Yourself. Maybe it's time to stop trying to justify your actions or convince those who are not supportive that you are on the right path. It would be ideal to have your child's other parent be a strong advocate at your side, but if that is not going to happen, perhaps it's easier to focus your energies elsewhere. You will be able to find allies in your support group, and they will point you in the direction of finding treatment. There's nothing wrong with you deciding to take full responsibility for trying to solve this problem yourself. It might not be what you signed up for, but maybe it has to be that way.

3. Change the Topic. If the unsupportive parent or extended family members starts lecturing and nagging, do your best to change the topic. Conversations can be fairly easy to redirect. Try phrases such as, "That's an interesting idea," or "Hadn't thought of that," then bring up a different topic. If the individual demands a response, tell him or her that you will get back with answers just as soon as they are available.

4. Don't Engage. There's no point in trying to defend yourself against a bully. All it does is deplete the energy that you need to apply elsewhere. If you find yourself beginning a sentence with,"That's not true..." or something similar, you're headed in the wrong direction. "I'll think that over," may be a better response. Your goal is to end the conversation as quickly as possible and move on to more important things.

5. Redouble Your Efforts to Find a Supportive Treatment Provider. Stop visiting doctors who tell you that you are wrong when your heart knows you're right. You know that PANDAS is a viable disorder. You know how unlikely it is that poor parenting is the cause of *any* mental health disorder. If a provider tells you there is no such thing as PANDAS or blames your parenting skills as the reason for your child's illness, my advice is don't walk away, run.

6. Look to Your Friends. You only need one solid person as an ally. It would be preferable to have a family network cheering you on, but sometimes life doesn't work that way. If you have friends to support you, you can do this. Truly, you just need one good friend who will be there for you at every step of the way. I had my friend Chris. She helped me to research and encouraged me when it seemed hopeless. There is someone like that for you; you just need to find that person. A number of moms turn up at my readings with their support person. Quite often that person is not a relative, but a close friend.

7. Take a Short Trip. Go visit a friend for an overnight and leave your child with family members. I know it might be torturous because of the worry, but as long as your child will be safe, it might be a good experiment. If unsupportive family members get a full dose of PANDAS parenting, they might change their tune. While you are away, try to rest up and enjoy the break.

Sibling Issues

As is true with any major disease, the needs of a sick family member will dominate the household. A sick child places tremendous strain on family members and on their relationships with each other. We all feel inadequate when our kids are seriously ill because, try as we might, we can't make it better. We'd change places with them in an instant, but instead are forced to watch as they suffer. Sometimes all that anger, frustration, and hopelessness comes out sideways. We become impatient and short-tempered with the people around us, particularly those with whom we are closest. As is true in any strained family situation, the children often act out all the underlying tension in their own unique ways. They can be angry and resentful, take on the role of caregiver, or withdraw into a shell.

Siblings are in a difficult spot. They feel badly for the sick child, but often equally (if not mostly) badly for themselves. From their perspective, this is something that is happening to them just as much as it is happening to the sick sibling. Their friends don't have siblings who tic, jerk, spin, and moan. Why did this have to happen to them? They may be resentful and feel they are getting the short end of the stick because the ill child always comes first. Simultaneously, they may be plagued by guilt for feeling that way. They may silently wonder if it was something they did or said that caused this to happen. If the parents are fighting over the illness and blaming one another, there are more reasons to resent the sick child. As far as they are concerned, everything was just fine before the sibling became sick.

Adolescents

> *Dear Beth,*
> *My PANDAS boy is my middle child. He was just diagnosed after months of agony. My oldest daughter (thirteen) insisted he was doing it all for attention. We just had the whole family tested for strep. It turns out she's the carrier. Now she's even more furious, accusing us of blaming her for his PANDAS (which we're not). Any advice?*
> *Teenage Tension*

Dear Tension,

I think she's horrified by her own behavior, so it's easier for her to paint you as the bad guy. I'd do a lot of general talking about people making mistakes. You might tell her about a few you've made and how tough it was to forgive yourself. If you verbalize it, perhaps she'll be able to think it through and begin to forgive herself. The next time she starts blaming, you can reference the earlier conversation and suggest that forgiving herself might be a better approach.

Beth

Adolescent siblings are especially tough. Adolescence is not a particularly empathetic time of life. It's usually a touchy time without adding the jumble of emotions brought about by a sick sibling. Adolescents are beginning to feel self-sufficient. They're on a trajectory toward greatness and independence. Everyone other than their friends either doesn't get it or is holding them back. Remember those feelings? Many adolescents feel they are already unfairly burdened with parents who do not understand them. It's a time of urgently wanting everything to move forward into adulthood, and the sick sibling is a big inconvenience. Most things in an adolescent's world tend to revolve around what they need and want at any given moment. As difficult as many adolescents think their lives already are, thrusting a sick sibling into the middle makes the family dynamic even more treacherous to negotiate. To top it off, there may be the underlying suspicion that the sick child is doing this for attention because "she was fine before!"

Don't be upset if your adolescent isn't helpful or understanding. It's not an empathetic time of life.

Even though all your energy is depleted and you're holding it together by a thread, you have to remember that family rifts can last a lifetime, so be very careful. Adolescents need you, too. They can't go through the ordinary pull and tug of growth if you're completely unavailable. They need to be able to tell you about the monumental problems in their lives (that honestly may not amount to much in the greater scheme of things), and you need to at least pretend you think those problems are important. If you are completely unavailable to them, you may lose them entirely. Don't let PANDAS steal another one from you.

Reach into that deep reservoir of parental patience, remember how cute they were when they were little, and validate their feelings. Instead of pointing out how unreasonable they're being, bite your tongue and tell them you understand how hard this is for them. Add in how hard it is for you, too, and everyone in the family especially the child who is sick. If they happen to do something slightly helpful or kind, make a big deal out of it. If there is a way to do something special with them, to make them feel that they are the center of your universe, it might help. Find something good to say about them every day. Adolescence is genuinely a time of struggle, and what you perceive as a minor glitch can be huge to an

Find one positive thing to say about your sick child's adolescent sibling every day.

adolescent. There are times when you will need to call the adolescent to task, but try to find an equal number of times when you can tap in to the generous side of their emerging selves. It's hard work, but someday PANDAS will be over. You don't want your family left permanently disrupted by what will eventually have been a rough patch you went through. Under no circumstances, however, may any sibling be unkind to the sick child.

Younger Siblings

> *Dear Beth,*
> *My oldest son has PANDAS with lots of OCD. The other day my youngest, who is eight, ran into the room and burst into tears saying, "Mom, I just washed my hands twice. Maybe I've got it!" Do you have any advice for me?*
> *Scared Sibling's Mom*

> *Dear Sib's Mom*
> *I think you need to make sure to spend separate sweet time with your littlest. He must be so scared right now.*
> *Beth*

Younger siblings present different considerations. The older ones had the benefit of years of your attention and are probably willing to aggressively vocalize the unfair twist of fate. The younger ones may simply get lost in the chaos. They may quietly withdraw in an effort to be non-demanding. They may start imitating the sick child's behaviors so that they, too, catch your attention. They may feel scared that they will come down with the illness or feel guilty that they are well. Chances are your home has become a very sad place to be, and they feel it. Their friends can't come to play. It's hard to get them where they need to go. Fighting among parents and adolescent siblings may cause the littlest ones to choose to fade into the background.

> *Find one-on-one time to spend with your sick child's younger siblings. They need you. Don't let them get lost.*

Those years never come back. Try to find some special time to spend with the younger siblings and treasure every special moment. At the same time, insulate them as much as possible from your concerns. Try to keep their lives moving along as if one child were not desperately ill. Arrange play dates for them at other's houses. Ask those other parents if they'll help you out by driving. Reassure the younger siblings that they do not need to worry, that you are the grown up and taking care of everything. The last thing you want is young children burdened with feeling responsible for taking care of the grown ups or siblings in their lives.

Extended Family and Friends

> Dear Beth,
>
> *I seem to be hitting a brick wall holding our lives together. Constance (eleven) diagnosed PANDAS, Jeffrey (eight) PANDAS prone, and Stevey (six) PANDAS prone are under treatment. Do you have any motherly advice for how to keep sane? I know you were raising your three boys and juggling a career as Sammy became ill and eventually better. I kind of feel like I am going to fall apart at any minute... knowing you got through it helps, but I still feel like I am falling short...*
>
> *Falling*

Dear Falling,
I felt like that all the time. It was so very hard, and the guilt was
unbearable. Try to take it one day at a time, remind yourself that
you're doing your best under incredibly difficult circumstances. Most
important, be willing to ask for help.
Beth

We would all like to be "superparents" and handle everything at all times with incredible skill. That's a wonderful goal. It means never getting upset with our children, managing to be in two places at once, and not forgetting to take the list along when you go grocery shopping. PANDAS, however, isn't just one more thing to take care of. It may be the biggest challenge of your life, and you want to come through this still standing with your sanity intact. To get help, you have to be able to ask for it or respond to the offers made by others, and that means you must first be willing to talk about what is going on at home. If you are embarrassed to share the facts, or worried about other people's reactions, then you won't be able to get help. If you are still blaming yourself, then you will be reluctant to open yourself up to the help you need. If a drunk driver smashed into your car, sharing the story wouldn't be an issue, and that's how you need to think of PANDAS. It's something that happened to you, not something you caused. You may want to be prudent about what you say to whom, but you have to speak up and use your voice.

I thought I did a good job of using my voice, but apparently I didn't do as well as I thought. Many of my friends were shocked when they read *Saving Sammy.* They had no idea how truly dark and hopeless our lives had become. I was fortunate because I had a large network of people on whom I knew I could rely for help. I had friends who would look after my youngest. I had friends who would drive Sammy to the few appointments that I didn't need to attend. I had friends and family whom I could call whenever I hit the breaking point. You need those same supports. If you don't have a similar network then you need to create one. Speak with your neighbors. Let your children's teachers know what's going on. If it's too hard to discuss it without breaking down, maybe you can simply hand them a copy of *Saving Sammy* and say, "This is what we're going through, and I need help."

Once you make people aware of what's happening, many will ask, "What can I do to help?" It will be best if you have an answer ready.

> 👉
> *Make a list of all the things that would make things easier for you. That way you'll be ready to respond when people ask what they can do to help. Work up the courage to reach out and ask for what you need.*

When one of my friends was struck with a serious illness, she printed a detailed list of the things she needed: groceries, prepared foods, toiletries, household items, even her favorite take-out meals. When someone asked her, "What can I do to help?" she gave that person the list. As a first step, put your own list together. Make it a wish list. Take a look around your home and write down everything that could help make your life a little easier. Perhaps it is as simple as watching your child for just a bit so you can get out for a short walk. It might make a big difference if someone would go grocery shopping for you, help you clean your kitchen, do your laundry once, take items to the recycling center, drive your youngest to soccer, or bring over a spaghetti dinner. It might feel good if someone would just stop by to talk and share a cup of coffee. Write down every single thing that might help, then hang it on your refrigerator or type it into your smart phone. When someone asks how he or she might help, you'll be ready with an answer. If your needs are big, if you are in need of food for example, you might talk to someone at a religious or community organization. If you need help with medicine, the manufacturers sometimes have sections on their websites where patients can e-mail to ask for help. If you cannot find anything on the website, pick up the telephone and call.

Asking for help is something that gets easier. And remember that most people like to help. It makes them feel good.

Thoughts About Help from a PANDAS Mom (see Callie's Story in chapter 13, "Hospitalization")

"In the beginning, when Callie first got sick, I pushed away all attempts to help. The inner Wonder Woman in me felt I could still take care of our family. When that failed, the strain I felt from worrying and caring for our sick child was multiplied by guilt for the siblings I was unable to properly care for. My husband was working overtime to keep up with the medical bills. I was at the hospital with Callie. Our other two girls were coming home to an empty house with no dinner. When I saw my pride was making my other children suffer, I decided I needed to call on those who had offered to help. I had friends stop by to check on my kids and bring them dinner. They arranged rides to practice and left muffins and other goodies at my door with little notes. I can't tell you how much this meant to all of us, not to mention the person who helped. People in your life genuinely want to help when tragedy strikes, and they feel inadequate until you give them a task. Allow them to help. You will feel better, and they will feel better, too."

SUMMING IT UP

Sometimes the people who we wish most would be there for us, cannot or will not be willing to help. You have two choices. You can either keep banging your head up against the brick wall of unsupportive people, or you accept it as a fact and find different supports. Other parents who have lived through your journey may be the best people to offer you emotional support and medical guidance; seek them out. Your other children may feel this has happened to them as much as to their sick sibling. Find the time and patience to help them through their emotions. When people do offer to help, be ready to accept their generosity. Be prepared to let them know what would mean the most to you—and don't forget to say thank you.

BIG IDEAS FROM CHAPTER TWELVE

❑ Moms most often take the lead in making health-care decisions for their family members.

❑ Doctors and the greater medical community are not always right.

❑ Poor parenting and inadequate discipline are not the cause of your child's behaviors.

❑ Other family members do not have the power to cure your PANDAS child's behavioral problems.

❑ Support can be found outside of your immediate family members.

❑ Siblings of the PANDAS child still need your attention, love, and reassurance even when they are difficult.

❑ Ask for help when you need it.

❑ Accept help from those who offer.

❑ Say thank you.

❑ Try to take things one day at a time and remind yourself that one day this will all be over.

Hospitalization

Dear Beth,

Thank you for sharing your story about Sammy. As I write this, my twelve-year-old son is in the other room compulsively bouncing his small super ball and occasionally clearing his throat. He was diagnosed with OCD four years ago and our lives have been turned upside down ever since. For the past three years, winter and spring is when his anxiety/OCD, headaches, and stomach pain become unmanageable, he is not able to attend school or even leave the house much. His 800 strep titer was dismissed by a neurologist. A child psychiatrist put him on Zoloft. Initially it helped. He started changing his clothes and showering again, but after a few months it stopped working, and he was a zombie. On Prozac he went absolutely mad. I was afraid he would hurt himself or his little brother so I called a local mental health hospital for help. Hearing the screams and my sobs they sent the police and my son (then nine) was arrested. I wanted him taken to a hospital. They took him to the juvenile detention center. I was able to go get him and bring him home after a couple hours, but it was the absolute worst day of our lives. When I read Saving Sammy, I felt like I was reading about our lives. I don't want to get my hopes up, but I made an appointment with one of the doctors from your list. We are seeing him next week. I am going to do what you did and write his history for the doctor to read before we see him. I just hope it's not too late.

Never Giving Up

When PANDAS children are not diagnosed and/or appropriately treated, their behaviors grow ever more concerning. Sometimes, the child slowly deteriorates such as when a refusal to eat becomes a life-threatening condition. Other times, there may be an unmanageable and dangerous explosion of behaviors that places the child and others at risk. In extreme cases, PANDAS children have tried to jump from moving cars, run away, and threatened to kill or hurt themselves or others. It's possible the psychotropic medications they're taking are increasing the behaviors. Or perhaps they have stopped responding to whatever medication has been prescribed. For whatever reason, you may feel the situation has become beyond your ability to handle. At that point, although you have tried your very best, the decision may be made to take the child to the hospital.

While some cases become very dangerous overnight, more often the parents and caregivers have watched a progressive slide downward or a continuing escalation. If you find yourself wondering how much longer you will be able to manage the situation, do some early exploring and planning in case your child ultimately needs hospitalization. Some of the questions to consider are:

- ❑ What does the hospital have to offer?
- ❑ Is there a hospital in your area that has a better reputation than others for working with children in difficult situations?
- ❑ Does your child's doctor think one hospital is better than another?
- ❑ What coverage does your insurance company offer and are there referrals that will need to be made?
- ❑ Who will watch your other children while you are at the hospital with your PANDAS child?

You want to avoid hospitalization unless it is a step that you absolutely must take, but sometimes the situation is so serious that you do not have a choice. This chapter describes what you can expect if you eventually decide that hospitalization is your only option. It describes emergency medicine, explains how an emergency department of one city hospital approaches a child in crisis, and shares the perspective of a parent who lived the ordeal. Becoming familiar in advance will help make a difficult situation less traumatic for everyone involved.

Unfortunately, due to the heartbreaking experience of some parents, this chapter will open with a primer on child welfare.

A Word of Caution: The Child Welfare System

Child protection cases generally come to the attention of the public when a particularly horrendous case is reported by the news media. State officials come under the spotlight for failing to step in and use their power to have a horribly abused child removed from his or her caregiver. When the media attempts to probe, state officials refuse to comment, citing the confidentiality of child protection matters. Unfortunately, when a powerful state agency is permitted to operate in secret, abuse is likely to occur within the agency itself. Coupled with the belligerence of the medical community, PANDAS parents and children are vulnerable to being caught in the vortex and forced to keep silent about it.

By way of background, the legislature of each state has enacted laws about confidentiality in matters of child abuse. The purpose of those laws is to protect the privacy of abused children. As a society, we have grown to believe that children should be sheltered. We don't want the name of a sexually abused minor spread through the press. We want that child's identity protected so the child has an opportunity to quietly heal and recover. What has happened in the PANDAS cases, though, is a perversion of that intent. Under the guise of protecting children, the laws are invoked to keep secret the actions of the hospital and the state. Protecting the hospital and state from scrutiny was never the legislative intent, but these laws are being regularly invoked as a shield. For that reason, it is important for you to understand the basics of the system and to do your homework on where you will take your child for treatment.

Under the child welfare systems of each state, certain individuals are designated as "mandated reporters." A mandated reporter must notify state authorities when he or she suspects child abuse or neglect. Teachers are mandated reporters and so are health-care professionals. If they think a child is being abused, they have no choice but to report it. So, for example, if a child is brought to the ER with several broken bones and there is no good explanation for what happened, the doctor is obligated to file a report of suspected child abuse. The state investigates the report and then makes a determination of whether the child has been abused. Usually the reporters are well intentioned. But filing a report with child protective services can also be used as a weapon, and it has been—against the parents of PANDAS children.

You cannot assume that hospitals are always staffed with well-meaning treatment providers doing whatever they can to help. Some are arrogant and vicious. In some circumstances, nonbelieving hospitals and doctors have reported caring, attentive parents for neglect and abuse of their PANDAS children even though the parents are following the advice of treating physicians. Those hospitals and doctors have caused parents to lose custody of children because it is their position that PANDAS does not exist. Their goal is to prove you wrong and—perhaps more important to them—your doctors wrong, too. Mark my words, that type of hospital will cause the state to take your child. The legal battle it will wage while hiding in the state's shadow will be long and unrelenting. You will be accused of atrocities. Every aspect of your life will be dissected by uninformed social workers. You will be skewered for challenging doctors who insist that your child's condition is purely psychiatric although you have clear evidence of an infectious basis.

I know this to be true because I have personally handled legal cases for parents involving one of the biggest hospitals in Boston.

It's imperative that you only bring your child to a PANDAS-friendly hospital. I know how scary this sounds, but you don't want to end up at a place that will immediately cut off your child's antibiotics, call in the hospital's social worker, and report you to state authorities. You don't want to be among those well-meaning parents who have explained to hospital staff how long it took them to find the right treatment, and how many doctors it took to find the right one, only to hear those words twisted and used in accusations of "doctor shopping" or "seeing multiple providers." You don't want to be...

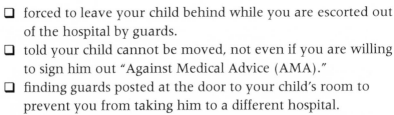

- ❏ forced to leave your child behind while you are escorted out of the hospital by guards.
- ❏ told your child cannot be moved, not even if you are willing to sign him out "Against Medical Advice (AMA)."
- ❏ finding guards posted at the door to your child's room to prevent you from taking him to a different hospital.
- ❏ threatened with losing custody of your child if you do not immediately and "voluntarily" sign the child into the hospital's locked psychiatric unit.

❑ given notice at 5PM to attend an emergency court hearing at 9AM the next morning where you may lose custody of your child and all rights to direct medical treatment.

These are real life situations so I implore you to figure out in advance where it is safe for you to take your child if an emergency situation arises. Do not make the mistake of assuming that a "children's hospital" will be a safe choice; they can be among the worst. As a rule of thumb, I would recommend staying away from any children's hospital that has its own psychiatric wing. Preferably, you want to enter a PANDAS-friendly hospital under the protective eye of a caring physician who has privileges (the right to practice medicine) at that hospital. Do your research and don't make assumptions. Contact other parents through PANDAS support groups to learn about their experiences with different hospitals

If you find yourself in one of the situations mentioned above, you must immediately find an attorney who is experienced in child protection law and can help get your child out before things deteriorate further. Child protection law is a separate specialty; it is not family law. Frankly, you might want to have a good attorney lined up in advance just in case things start to take a disturbing turn.

The balance of this chapter assumes that you are working with a reasonable hospital, not one intent on taking your child to justify its position that PANDAS does not exist.

Emergency Medicine

Children in crisis arrive at the ER of local, regional, and city hospitals by ambulance, police transport, or by car if their parents are able to bring them. The ER is a busy place. Patients go there because they need immediate treatment. ER doctors are fully trained to provide critical care for victims of heart attacks and traumatic injuries from car crashes, violent crimes, or serious accidents. They can set broken bones and assess head concussions. And the ER has recently become the front line for medical care of uninsured patients, often treating routine ailments such as pediatric ear infections.

FACT: The ER does not offer long-term solutions to mental health ailments or behavioral disorders.

But while the ER doctors and others there will want to help your child, it is not a place that will offer you solutions for mental health and behavioral disorders.

What Happens at the ER? What happens at the ER will depend upon the degree of your child's behaviors. If your child's refusal to eat has placed her in a life-threatening condition, she will be admitted to the hospital. But if the symptoms are dangerous behaviors, there will be a different path. In the case of a highly agitated child, the ER will have two goals: how to stabilize the patient and where will it be best for him to go when he's discharged? Because mental health is not an area of expertise for ER physicians, the hospital will try to contact your child's doctor or find a mental health professional to help them.

FACT:
If you decide to take your child home before the doctors think he is ready, you may need to sign a form acknowledging that you are making that decision "against medical advice."

What if a Child is Violent? If you bring your child to the ER because he is dangerously out of control, and if the staff is not successful in calming him, he may be restrained in a physical hold and given a shot of medication to help calm or sedate him. Depending upon the level of danger, the police might even be called. If you visit a major city hospital, there may be a separate wing for psychiatric patients that is locked off from the rest of the ER. Depending upon your child's age, size, and behaviors, he might be placed in that wing, where staff may observe him from behind large glass panels. Once the child is stabilized, then a decision has to be made about what to do next. You might want to take your child home, but the hospital may be reluctant to release him back to your care if it feels your child may be a danger to himself or others. In that case, the goal will be to find an available bed for inpatient treatment based on an assessment that recommends what is appropriate. If you remain determined to take your child home, you may need to acknowledge in writing that you are doing so "against medical advice."

How Is a Child Assessed for Further Treatment? The size of the hospital where you visit the ER will often determine how your child is assessed for further treatment. At a large teaching hospital, there will be residents and attending physicians available to help patients who have mental health and behavioral disorders. Smaller community hospitals will probably need to call an outside provider such as a child psychiatrist or a mental health organization to make the assessment. Whether your child has private or state health insurance may also be a factor in how the assessment takes place.

How Long Will the Child Be at the ER? Your child will be at the ER only until he is stabilized and assessed, then he will be admitted or discharged either to home or another facility. Due to the structure of our Medicaid system, children are usually not treated in the "psych wing" of a general hospital. Instead, free-standing hospitals offer inpatient psychiatric services for children. If the assessment indicates that your child is not safe to go home, then while your child stabilizes in the ER, hospital staff will begin to explore where there may be an available bed at an inpatient facility. Due to the shortage of beds, staff may need to explore out-of-state options. Once the bed is located, your child may have to be transported by ambulance to his new placement.

Why Might a Hospital Social Worker Become Involved? Child welfare is of particular concern at the ER because it is often where abused children are brought after they are injured. Whether the child has a burn or extreme behaviors, the ER team wants to do the best they can to make sure the child is safe. When they feel circumstances warrant a closer look, they will contact the appropriate state authorities such as the police or your state's bureau of child welfare. If a PANDAS child ends up in the emergency room screaming, violent, and making threats, there will be reasonable concerns about whether something is happening at home that might cause those behaviors. For that reason, the hospital's social worker may meet with you to gain a better understanding. If you are approached due to those concerns, don't be defensive or surprised. Answer the questions as best you can while recognizing that most are genuinely looking out for your child's welfare. The hospital probably does not know about PANDAS. If the social worker appears receptive, perhaps you can help to educate him or her as part of the process; but keep your antennae up. If the hospital wants to accuse you of neglect or abuse, what you say to the social worker may be used against you.

Items to Bring to the ER. If you must take your child to the ER, there are some things you will want to bring along. If you anticipate that hospitalization is a step you may need to take, I recommend that you gather the items ahead of time. Drop them into a bag that you can grab if you are in a hurry. The bag should have:

- ❑ A list of all your child's doctors together with their contact information and areas of expertise.
- ❑ The names and dosages of all prescription medications, along with when the last dose was administered. Call your pharmacist to obtain a printout of medications. If you do not have the list ready at the time you go to the hospital, scoop up the prescription bottles and bring them along.
- ❑ A copy of your health insurance card.
- ❑ A fresh set of clothing for you child.
- ❑ A favorite book or other item for your child.

Visits to the ER take a long time, so expect to wait. Bringing something along to occupy your own time will prove wise. In May of 2012, an article in the Annals of Emergency Medicine reported that psychiatric patients spent more than eleven hours in the ER on average when seeking care.

☛

Get a bag ready "just in case" that contains:

- *Physician contact information*
- *Prescription medications and dosages*
- *Health insurance card*
- *Extra clothes*
- *Comfort items*

The Hospital's Viewpoint

For guidance in describing emergency admission and treatment from the hospital's point of view, I spoke with Michael Baumann, MD, head of emergency medicine for Maine Medical Center (MMC) in Portland. I wanted to find out what would happen if a PANDAS child were brought to that hospital's ER in crisis. The Emergency Department at MMC is extremely busy, with 65,000 visits per year. This is comparable to the number of visits at ERs in major hospitals in Boston and New York City. MMC is a teaching hospital so there are resident physicians on staff, as well as attending physicians, psychiatrists, social workers, nurses, and physician assistants. And the emergency department is divided into different sections. There is a large area with rooms for all emergencies, but pediatrics, psychiatry, and critical care have their own separate sections. While your experience at a smaller community hospital will be somewhat different, the general principles will be the same.

What Happens First? The first step will be a visit to triage. *Triage* is the process of having a nurse determine the priority of a patient's needs so that the sickest patients will be seen more quickly than those who can wait. Triage determines when your child will be seen and, if the hospital has separate treatment areas, where she will be evaluated. After triage and room placement, patients with behavioral concerns are seen by the medical staff to be "medically cleared."

What Is Medical Clearance? For a child, "medical clearance" means making sure the child did not ingest any drugs and that vital signs are normal. Questions will be asked of the parents and there will be a physical exam to determine, for example, whether the child has a fever. Dr. Baumann contrasted medical clearance for a child with clearance for an older patient. In an older patient, the ER looks not only for drug effects and abnormal vital signs, but also for an infection. This is because infections are recognized as a frequent cause of a change in an older patient's behavior. For children, though, that last step—the one where infection is ruled out—is usually not taken if the child appears physically well upon examination. Instead, consistent with nationwide practice, the next step will be for a mental health provider to see the child.

> **FACT:**
> *When children are admitted to the ER with behavioral problems, they will not be tested for infections unless they show the typical physical symptoms (temperature, sore throat). For elderly patients exhibiting behavioral changes, an infection is always considered.*

Who Does the Mental Health Assessment? The mental health provider will be responsible for assessing your child's condition and needs. Which mental health provider will evaluate your child depends to some degree on your health insurance coverage. Some insurance providers have contracted with specific mental health organizations to do the assessments on their insureds. If the agency your insurer has contracted with has no one available when the assessment is needed, MMC will perform the assessment itself. Either way, the resulting assessment is quite lengthy.

What Happens After the Assessment? The assessment will make recommendations for what should happen next. The assessment will evaluate if the child is stable enough to go home and whether the home appears to be safe. If the child or home is unsafe, then the assessment will recommend the care that the assessor feels will be best for the child. This may be psychiatric hospitalization or it may be a crisis center. A crisis center is an interim step that offers short-term stays for children pending further decisions about what to do next. There is always a shortage of available inpatient beds and, if your child requires that level of care, she will have to go to the facility where there is an opening. For example, if the child is in crisis at a hospital in southern Maine, but the only available bed is at Acadia Hospital in Bangor (three hours away) that is where the child will go. This process of finding a bed can take many additional hours, so be prepared to wait.

Psychiatric Hospitalization

> *Dear Beth,*
> *This summer our teenage grandson spent three weeks in the psychiatric unit at our local hospital. His strep titer was over 800, and he was diagnosed as having PANDAS. He was put on psychotropic meds and also penicillin. Shortly after receiving penicillin his OCD symptoms improved immensely. A little later he developed depression and some of his OCD symptoms returned. After reading Saving Sammy our daughter encouraged the doctor to put him on Augmentin. During the time he was on Augmentin he seemed much better, but the doctor then gave him another antibiotic that the doctor said was safer to take for a longer period of time. He's now so severely depressed that he's in a residential program. The hospital psychiatrist says she has read*

a lot about PANDAS. She doesn't feel the long-term antibiotics is the answer so they won't give them to him. We are at our wits end. His anxiety is so severe he often can't use the bathroom. Is there any way you can help us?
    A Grieving Grandmother

Dear Grieving Grandmother,
It sounds as if the psychiatrist is well intentioned, but lacks any practical experience in treating PANDAS. Please find out if she will speak with me by telephone.
    Beth

We would like to think that a local psychiatric hospital (or even a crisis center) will be able to offer the best treatment. Unfortunately that is not always the case, particularly for PANDAS. The hospital may not recognize the disorder and some are full of staunch nonbelievers. If your child is so ill that psychiatric hospitalization is recommended, it's best to look at this as a way to find stabilization and safety while you devote yourself to figuring out what to do next, and that should be to find a knowledgeable physician. Be prepared that some psychiatric hospitals can be quite difficult. I know how vulnerable you will feel at such a time, and I know parts of this will not be easy to read, but I would rather have you be prepared than surprised.

Whether your child ends up hospitalized or in a crisis center, you will not have open access to your child. Similar to a general hospital, there will be limited hours when you will be allowed to visit. During those hours, along with checking on how your child is doing, observe how other patients are being treated. Is the staff kind and supportive or are they confrontative and demeaning? I encourage you to notice

During visiting hours, make sure you observe how staff treat other patients. Are they being kind?

because that is how staff is treating your child when you are not there. If you are not comfortable with anything you see, go to the nurses' station and file a report.

You may also find that your child becomes aggressive when you visit. Keep in mind that children often manage to contain their behaviors for periods of time, then explode. They may feel safer to "let go" when you are around to protect them. But this may cause the hospital to wonder if you are the cause of your child's behaviors. Painful as it may be for you and your child, you may need to stop visiting for a day or so. Your child will not be able to contain herself for days. When she acts out during your absence, staff should recognize that you are not responsible for the outbursts.

Over the course of your child's stay, you will be asked to meet periodically with the child's treatment team. At these meetings, your child's history and her prescriptions will be reviewed. Medication adjustments will be explained and made, those which the hospital's doctor feels may help. Time will be spent discussing behavioral plans and—frankly—assessing whether something went wrong with your parenting. There may be six or seven people in these meetings: the medical director, the child psychiatrist, a nurse, the social worker, the clinician or therapist, and perhaps others. Many parents find these types of meetings intimidating because there are so many professionals in the room. If you feel yourself being blamed—subtly or directly—you need to speak up immediately. This is not a time to politely listen and wonder if maybe it is all your fault. You already know it's not your fault. If you try to make suggestions or offer input, and hear comments such as, "If you knew what was best for him, he wouldn't be here," you should tell the speaker that the remark is inappropriate and unprofessional and you will not be treated like that. Perhaps you might also ask, "Are you suggesting it's my fault that doctors have failed to adequately treat my child?"

The hospital's treatment team often has its own idea of what is happening in the child's life and may not be particularly receptive to hearing other points of view. If your child has PANDAS, you may face the additional challenge of team members having little knowledge of the disorder or perhaps being unwilling to acknowledge that it exists. If you've broached the subject of an infection-based mental health disorder, and the team tries to explain that

It's okay to stick up for yourself, but don't waste energy trying to convince people that PANDAS exists. Your only goal is to line up appropriate outside treatment and take your child home as soon as possible.

you are wrong or maybe enabling the child by making excuses for her behavior, don't put a lot of energy into defending yourself. Just state your position and remind them that you are the one who knows your child best. They have known her only for a short time under the worst of circumstances.

If you have a good relationship with your child's school, you might want to invite someone from the school to attend the team meeting. If school personnel cannot attend in person, attendance by speakerphone is an option. The school may have valuable input regarding schooling that may take place in the hospital, it may be familiar with the development of your child's condition, and it may offer support for the perspective that whatever is going on is not your fault should the hospital be trying to assess blame.

When your child is well enough to leave the hospital, there will be a final discharge meeting with the treatment team. Your personal goal should be to have the appropriate providers lined up to work with your child immediately upon discharge.

> *Dear Beth,*
>
> *After struggling for years my daughter is, once again, in our local psychiatric hospital. This is her fourth psychiatric hospitalization in six years. She has never tested positive for group A strep, but we suspected PANDAS because it all happened so suddenly when she was eight. Her violence has come and gone over the years, but now it's back and she's even hitting herself hundreds of times a day. Do you have any ideas for us?*
>
> *Sad and Sorry*

> *Dear Sad and Sorry,*
>
> *Has she ever been tested for mycoplasma or Lyme?*
>
> *Beth*

> *Dear Beth,*
>
> *That was it! Both tests came back positive!*
>
> *No Longer Sad and Sorry*

Callie's Story: Hospitalization/Outpatient Clinic

There are a number of behavioral clinics around the country devoted to addressing targeted behavioral issues such as obsessive-compulsive and eating disorders. While many are engaged in treating the behavioral symptoms of the disorders, most are not addressing the underlying infection that is the root cause; that failure almost cost one little girl her life.

Callie was an adorable ten-year-old who liked to play with her two sisters, earn badges with her Girl Scout troop, and collect money for charities. Callie's mom took her to the pediatrician because she had been sick with a really bad cold and sore throat. Callie had also started weighing herself ten times a day and jumping. Callie was very active on her swim team and thin. Weight and appearance never mattered much to Callie; she was more of a tomboy who enjoyed climbing trees and searching for frogs with the neighborhood boys. At the appointment, because of the significance of the weight loss issue, the pediatrician focused only on that, ignoring the cold and sore throat that Callie's mom had pointed out. The pediatrician made an immediate referral to an eating disorder clinic that was associated with a hospital in Portland, Oregon. Callie's family arrived at the clinic, thinking they would have a simple screening and fact-gathering interview. Things took a very different turn when Callie's physical exam detected a low body temperature and heart beat, along with corresponding problems with her blood pressure. Those conditions can be signs of potential fatality for a child. She was admitted to the hospital.

Upon admission, one of the nurses asked if Callie had been sick lately. Callie's mother related the bad sore throat, persistent cough, and nonstop cold that she had described to the pediatrician. The nurse also wanted to know if her behavior was out of character, or if she'd always been concerned about her weight. When Callie's mother said it was completely out of character, that her daughter had never cared about her weight before, the nurse suggested testing Callie's blood for strep and asked her if she had heard of PANDAS. Callie's mom, shell-shocked from what was unfolding, remembers asking, "Do you mean the bear?" The nurse then explained that some people thought strep could cause a behavioral reaction. When the test came back with an elevated titer, the doctor from the eating disorder clinic offered to put Callie on five days of antibiotics, saying some people believe that may help, and left the decision to Callie's parents. Callie's mom remembers thinking, "If it may help, why wouldn't we want to do it?" She immediately gave the okay.

Callie had to stay in the hospital for one week because of the concerns about her blood pressure and heart. At times, it was only beating 35 times a minute. After a few days, Callie was willing to eat. She was discharged with the understanding that she would attend the affiliated eating disorder clinic. The antibiotics were discontinued, psychotropic medications were introduced, and Callie began attending the eating disorder program at the clinic.

As time passed, Callie's mom became increasingly concerned about the approach of the program. Most of the girls were teenagers, and there were aspects of humiliation. Callie was forced to eat any crumbs that fell off her plate, and she was watched as she used the bathroom. Callie's mother recalled that, "Callie was treated as if she were a sixteen-year-old who had looked at *Vogue* magazine and wanted a different figure." During parents' night at the clinic, Callie's mom could not find a common thread between her story and those of the other families. She also felt Callie was gaining an education about things the little girl had never heard of before such as bulimia. Callie herself hated the clinic. One day she announced that she would never go there again, and that she was not going to eat anymore. Then she tried to run away.

The eating clinic said that because Callie was a flight risk, she needed to return to the hospital. This time she was admitted to the behavioral health unit. Some of the patients in the unit had tried to kill themselves. Her backpack was searched and shoelaces and belts removed, even the framed picture of her family because it was glass. While she was there she learned about cutting and other dysfunctional behaviors. A "cutter" is a patient who repeatedly slices his or her skin just enough to draw blood. Callie did eat while she was there, prompting the clinic doctor to say she did not have an eating disorder. Despite that, when she was released from the hospital's behavioral health unit, the eating disorder clinic wanted her back. Callie's mom refused because she did not think they understood what Callie needed. She took Callie home, and they decided they would try to fight this on their own.

Callie was happy to be back at school and even thrived for a few days, but then she started eating less and less at home. Her family worried as her knees, lips, and fingers turned purple, and she grew weaker by the day. Callie's mom took her to the emergency room. She was given an IV, but the hospital wouldn't admit her because she had been diagnosed with an eating disorder so they wanted her at the clinic. Callie's mom did not want the eating disorder clinic in charge of her care again. Callie cried as they turned her away. She screamed, "Can't you see I need help!" Then she wrapped the IV line around her neck in a feeble attempt to show her suicidal desperation.

A few days later, her parents took her to a different hospital, one not affiliated with the clinic that Callie hated. She was admitted immediately and blood work was run. Again, it disclosed that her strep titer was high. During the week that Callie was in the hospital, she received antibiotics. It was during this hospitalization that a friend of Callie's mom asked if she had heard of *Saving Sammy*. Propelled by what she learned from the book and e-mails she exchanged with me, she armed herself with additional research and insisted that Callie be placed on long-term antibiotics. The doctors were initially resistant, but Callie's mom prevailed. Callie was prescribed antibiotics for another three weeks. After a seven-day stay, Callie was discharged and went back to school with a daily nutrition plan she was to follow in an attempt to get her back to a healthy weight.

Weeks later when the antibiotic prescription ran out, Callie began to fall apart. She didn't want to eat again. She was suicidal. She was hitting her head against the wall, spinning, saying she wanted to go back in time, and raging that she was possessed. Callie's parents took her—kicking, screaming, and hissing like a cat— for admission to the behavioral mental health unit at the new hospital. Callie's dad, a police officer, is an ex-football player who is 6'2" and weighs 225 pounds. Callie weighed 49 pounds. She was so aggressive and wild that her father could only contain her by putting her in handcuffs. Once there, it took two orderlies to control her.

The hospital's psychiatrist recommended that she go back on antibiotics and to test the entire family for strep, including the dog. Callie's oldest sister tested positive although she was asymptomatic. The family dog showed up as a carrier. Both were treated. Callie's mom insisted that Callie remain on long-term antibiotics. As a precaution, the family home was scrubbed from top to bottom to help eliminate any lingering strep. Within two weeks, Callie was back at school, where she has remained and is doing well, with occasional flare-ups when she is exposed to strep.

In retrospect, Callie's mom feels her daughter was being reinfected every time she came home, which is why she always regressed. Callie and her two sisters share a bathroom, inadvertently grabbing each other's towels and toothbrushes. The dog kissed each of their faces every morning.

After Callie finally stabilized, her mom contacted the eating disorder clinic to let them know the story. She explained that although Callie had been hospitalized for an eating disorder, Callie didn't have an issue with body image. Callie had an infection. She needed antibiotics, not psychological reprogramming. Callie's mom told the clinic she felt that if they had been more aggressive and prescribed long-term antibiotics right away, her family might have been spared six months of trauma. The clinic was only partially receptive, not even replying after she sent over supportive research studies.

Callie's mom feels that if she had not stepped in and taken control of the situation, demanding long-term antibiotics, that Callie would be in an institution by now. Callie's occasional behavioral flare-ups can always be tied to an illness: either someone in the house is sick or there is strep at school. Callie is on a maintenance dose of antibiotics. When the behavioral symptoms crop up, the dose is doubled. Callie's mom still feels as if she's, "flying blind," with doctors who are somewhat supportive, but not totally on board.

SUMMING IT UP

There may come a point when your child's behaviors or condition are so dangerous that you must take him to the hospital. If it seems this may happen, you should screen hospitals carefully in advance to know which one will be the best PANDAS-friendly place for your child. If you end up at the ER, remember that it cannot offer you long-term solutions, but it will help stabilize your child. The ER will also assess whether the child is safe to go home or needs further hospitalization. Part of the assessment will be to inquire about the safety of your home, and this inquiry is born of child welfare concerns. If your child must be transferred to a crisis center or psychiatric hospital, keep in mind that it's rare to find one familiar with PANDAS. Use the time while your child is hospitalized to line up appropriate care and take him home as soon as possible. A psychiatric hospital can be a difficult place, and patients quickly learn unhealthy behaviors from one another, such as cutting.

What the doctor says:

"In 2010, I began noticing a prevalence of high ASO titers in teen-agers who engage in cutting and other non-suicidal self-injurious behaviors. I started tracking them and found that two-thirds of those patients had elevated titers."

Richard Livingston, MD

BIG IDEAS FROM CHAPTER THIRTEEN

- ❏ The child protection system sometimes becomes involved with PANDAS children so do some research and find out which hospitals are PANDAS-friendly.
- ❏ Take your child to the emergency department when he is a danger to himself or others.
- ❏ If you feel that visiting the ER is a step you may need to take, prepare in advance:
    know the best place to take your child
    pack a bag with the items you will need
    have insurance coverage figured out ahead of time
    line up someone to watch your other children
- ❏ Recognize the limitations of the ER; it does not offer long-term solutions for mental health disorders.
- ❏ The ER is concerned with child welfare and may express concerns about safety in your home.
- ❏ The goal of the ER team will be stabilization; in extreme cases this may involve physical restraint and sedation.

- ❏ Following stabilization, your child will be assessed to determine future needs.
- ❏ If the child is not well enough to go home, a referral may be made to a crisis unit or to a psychiatric hospital for inpatient treatment.
- ❏ Any period of hospitalization should be viewed as an opportunity for you to regroup and go about finding appropriate help for your child.

Residential Care

14

Dear Beth,

For any parents whose children need a residential program to overcome their behaviors, please recommend Rogers Memorial Hospital in Wisconsin. Our daughter went for six weeks and came back a changed individual. Almost 100 percent of her care was paid for by insurance and the results speak for themselves. Last year she was a school dropout who could not move from a couch. Now she's back and succeeding at an Ivy League. I can't say enough good things about Rogers.

Proud Papa

FACT:
Children with PANDAS may be placed in residential care when they need more intensive help overcoming their behaviors, or perhaps if they have been hospitalized and are not yet deemed safe enough to return home.

The conversation about residential care usually comes up in one of two ways. One situation is when your child is living at home and doing better with management of the infection, but his behaviors are still debilitating. He may need more intensive help than can be obtained from a therapist. The other is that your child has been hospitalized and, rather than send him home, the doctors want him discharged to a residential program. Either instance requires great care and thorough exploration before agreeing to a placement.

If your child is living at home, you will be able to control which program he enters. But if your child is being discharged from a hospital, you may have less influence and feel pressured to have your child go where the hospital recommends. As difficult as it may be, resist simply giving the "okay" to the hospital's suggestion. Hospital personnel do not necessarily know what will be right for your child. As responsible parents, we do not leave decisions about our children to third parties. Before you place your child in a residential program you must fully understand what the program has to offer and whether it is capable of meeting your child's needs. At a minimum, you need to speak with the people in charge of the program itself.

This chapter explains how residential programs are generally structured, outlines the issues to consider, offers you questions to ask before agreeing to a particular placement, and describes a well-respected residential program to give you a snapshot of what you want to find.

Residential Programs in General

Residential programs are generally managed by large, mental health organizations. Children who enter these programs are unable to maintain at home. Sometimes this is due to illness. Equally often, children enter a residential program because of the extreme behaviors they exhibit from being abused or neglected by caregivers. The program may be offered in an institutional setting, perhaps with a school on the program's grounds, or in private residences from which the children attend the local public school. The children in the program all live together, and usually two residents will share a bedroom. The programs are often staffed with twenty-somethings who are on their way to other careers.

If you feel you are asking too many questions, then the program you're considering probably isn't the right one for you.

Programs vary, but children in a typical residential setting are motivated by various rewards attached to targeted behavioral "levels." For example, a child on Level Five will have fewer privileges than a child who has achieved Level One. Depending upon the program, the residents may be responsible for various age-appropriate tasks associated with running a household. This may range from cleaning their own rooms and handling their own laundry, to helping with cooking and being assigned responsibility for cleaning the bathroom. These tasks are "life skills" that each resident is expected to demonstrate.

As basic as this criteria will sound, you want your child living in a program where the staff is kind and there is a true understanding of what your child is going through. For that reason, you must thoroughly research and understand the program you are considering. The atmosphere in many of these programs can be punitive; you want your child in a placement that encourages positive reinforcement. Unless a wealth of information is available about the intended program, you must personally visit and be ready to ask questions. This is not a time to be shy. If others are irritated by your questions, you should not wonder if something is wrong with your questions. Instead, you should wonder what is wrong with the program. You are entitled to all the information you need to make a good decision, so that you feel comfortable with where your child will be temporarily living. This means that a careful inquiry should be appreciated and the answers you receive should be responsive.

What to Do First

Ideally, the first step is to visit the program for a tour and to meet with the director. While on the tour, be a detective and observe everything around you.

- ❑ What is the atmosphere in the program?
- ❑ Is it positive or oppressive?
- ❑ What are the residents doing?
- ❑ Do they look happy and engaged?
- ❑ Are members of the staff interacting with or ignoring the residents?
- ❑ Does the person escorting you seem to genuinely care?

When you sit down to meet with the director, treat this as a job interview. You are attempting to determine whether this program can be hired to handle the task at hand. Ask the director to explain to you the disorder that best describes your child's symptoms such as OCD, anxiety, tics. If the director does not give you a good explanation then you need to find another program. You cannot risk having your child being treated as a discipline issue due to behaviors he cannot control. If you feel the disorder is adequately explained, then ask about PANDAS. If the director does not know anything about it or comes across as not believing that infections can trigger behavioral disorders, look elsewhere. It's tough enough to have your child living separately from you without fighting an uphill battle over what caused you to be at this juncture. If your instinct tells you this is not the right place, trust it. If you find yourself wanting to bolt from your chair and run to your car: be polite, thank them, and leave.

Assuming you believe you have found a kind and caring place that may be able to help your child, then you can move on to the other topics you need to cover. Below is a suggested checklist of topics and questions. Your discussion will probably lead to more questions so be sure to have your pen in hand.

Management of the Residence
- ❑ What is the schedule of daily life?
- ❑ What responsibilities will your child have?
- ❑ How often will your child come home?
- ❑ What are the limitations on visitation?
- ❑ What are the limitations on telephone calls?
- ❑ How are behavioral difficulties handled and documented?
- ❑ Who has access to any written documentation?
- ❑ Who will let you know if there is a problem with your child and how quickly will you be notified?
- ❑ How is a crisis situation handled?
- ❑ Which hospital emergency room is used by the program?
- ❑ Will you be immediately notified if your child is taken to the hospital?
- ❑ Who is responsible for notifying you?

Medical Concerns
- ❑ How will medicine be prescribed?
- ❑ How often will your child see a psychiatrist?
- ❑ Who is the psychiatrist?

- ❏ Is the psychiatrist part of the program or is the doctor's practice independent?
- ❏ Who is responsible for dispensing medication?
- ❏ Will staff be notified that your child is vulnerable to behavioral exacerbations when infections are present in other residents?

Therapy

- ❏ What type of therapy is offered to the residents?
- ❏ How often will your child see a therapist?
- ❏ Is the therapist trained in cognitive behavioral therapy?
- ❏ If so, what type of CBT—is it specifically designed to address your child's needs?
- ❏ Is the therapist on staff?
- ❏ What are the therapist's qualifications?

Review the chapter on CBT so you can quickly assess whether this program offers the therapy your child needs.

Other Residents

- ❏ What is the typical profile of the other residents?
- ❏ What is the typical length of stay in the program?
- ❏ Do most of the residents successfully transition home?
- ❏ How many of the residents have been in criminal trouble?
- ❏ What type of behaviors might your child learn from the other residents?

Staff

- ❏ What is the typical profile of the people who will look after your child?
- ❏ What type of qualifications must staff have to be hired?
- ❏ Is there an educational requirement?
- ❏ Are there ongoing training sessions for staff?
- ❏ What is the ratio of staff to residents?
- ❏ What is the typical staff turnover rate?
- ❏ Is a supervisor present on a daily basis?
- ❏ What happens if a resident clashes with a staff member?

Education

- ❏ How will your child's educational needs be met?
- ❏ Are there certified teachers on staff?
- ❏ If the children will attend public school, what is the reputation of the local school system?
- ❏ Will there be any coordination with the school system your child regularly attends when she is living with you?
- ❏ How will your child obtain any help that might be needed with completing homework?

Once you have completed the interview, then you must ask yourself a few questions. Do you trust the people you met? Do you feel this is a place that will understand your child? Is it a place where you want your child to live while she is not under your roof? Will she heal here?

I have often said that if Sammy had a different mother, he would have ended up in a residential program and constantly been on Level Five for something about his socks. As staff continued to insist that he either put on or take off his socks, ultimately there would have been a physical confrontation. He would have been placed in a four-point physical restraint (it's called a "hold") while socks were either forcibly pushed on or pulled off his feet. No one involved would have understood that he had an OCD rule about socks. He would have been humiliated, angry, and assaultive. The resultant aggression might have led to police involvement. A trip to the hospital emergency room, maybe even to a detention facility, might have followed.

So tread carefully. There are very few residential programs that will offer your PANDAS child what she needs: an understanding environment with the appropriate medical and therapeutic supports that will enable her to grow and flourish.

Rogers Memorial Hospital offers a program that exceeds the standard. By reading the below description, you will be able to identify whether the program you are considering offers at least most of what your child needs.

Rogers Memorial Hospital

Rogers Memorial Hospital is a freestanding, nonprofit hospital in Oconomowoc, Wisconsin. It is not managed by a large health-care organization. Rogers opened in 1907 and focuses on patients with behavioral disorders. The programs are designed to address OCD, anxiety, depression, eating disorders, bipolar disorder, and Asperger's. Patients are referred to Rogers by knowledgeable physicians across the country. It offers three programs for children and adolescents: inpatient, intensive outpatient (IOP), and residential. The inpatient unit focuses on safety and stabilization. It is a locked unit with twenty-two beds for children and adolescents who arrive in crisis and the usual stay is five to seven days. The IOP and residential programs are voluntary, so the children are far more stable than those who are inpatients. IOP is a month-long program. Patients participate in day treatment four hours per day, Monday through Thursdays, and must be at least twelve years old. For IOP, a parent must accompany any child under sixteen and the family resides in local lodging for the duration of the program.

The residential program for children and adolescents has been in operation since January 2003. In April of 2004, it doubled in capacity and added cognitive behavioral therapy. In 2012, the hospital completed construction on a new building for the Child and Adolescent Centers, which offers thirty-six beds for pediatric patients: twenty-four for adolescents and twelve for younger children. The children are grouped according to age. Patients eight to thirteen years old are in the Child Center. Older children are in the Adolescent Center. Although the upper age limit of children in the Child Center is thirteen, it's possible that a twelve- or thirteen-year-old might be treated in the Adolescent Center, depending upon the child's level of maturity. All the children live in a dormlike setting and, because participation is voluntary, it is not a locked unit or a program that uses physical restraint to compel compliance. The hospital maintains a consistent waiting list of about thirty prospective patients.

Peter Lake, MD, who is the hospital's medical director and child and adolescent psychiatrist, told me that Rogers is 100 percent supportive of PANDAS. Dr. Lake estimates that at least one patient a month arrives with OCD that was either triggered or exacerbated

What the doctor says:

"What I currently find exciting is a growing openness among my peers to consider PANDAS in the adult population."

Peter Lake, MD
Rogers Memorial Hospital

by strep. He believes it is appropriate to consider the possibility of PANDAS in almost every child who presents with OCD.

It is important to know that Rogers Memorial Hospital is not a "PANDAS hospital" that is full of "PANDAS doctors" who are experts in infection-triggered disorders; that hospital does not yet exist. What Rogers Memorial Hospital does offer is a residential program, which will address your child's behavioral symptoms while recognizing and being supportive of PANDAS. The hospital successfully treats PANDAS patients who have received or are receiving antibiotics or IV Ig, but continue to struggle behaviorally. Most are successfully treated with its comprehensive multimodal treatment approach of CBT/ERP, individual therapy, family involvement, group therapy, and medication adjustments. To help pinpoint the reasons for the hospital's treatment success, I spoke with Stephanie Eken, MD. She is the medical director of the Child Center at Rogers. Dr. Eken is board certified in child and adolescent psychiatry, adult psychiatry, and pediatrics. At any given time, there are ten children in the group she oversees.

Dr. Eken first credited the hospital's success to a great team, who are all dedicated to helping the children recover. She said the hospital's method of evidence-based treatment, coupled with the extensive training given to the behavioral specialists, results in a clear protocol. In short, there is no confusion as to the goal, or to the approach that will be used to reach that goal. Everyone is on the same page. The hospital's psychiatrists work hard to communicate with the child's parents and outpatient providers to ensure there is an accurate history of medication and behaviors. Rogers also has so many child psychiatrists on staff that the patient-physician ratio enables the doctors to see the patients frequently.

What the doctor says:

"In most states with residential programs, a psychiatrist only has to see the child once a month. At Rogers, each psychiatrist sees the patient three times a week, and tends to see them every day as part of the general milieu or social environment."

Stephanie Eken, MD
Rogers Memorial Hospital

"There are a lot of professional eyes on the child in a variety of settings and that's really helpful," Dr. Eken said. From 8AM until 5PM, the children are involved with psychiatrists, psychologists, family therapists, behavioral therapists, experiential therapists (ropes course, rock wall, boating, games such as capture the flag), residential counselors, nurses, and teachers. The generous staff-patient ratio enables each of these persons to be invested in the child's recovery, with the time to focus on what the child needs. The daytime ratio of staff to patients is two or three to each patient. At night, the ratio is four patients to one staff member.

The typical stay at Rogers is six to eight weeks. The first week is usually devoted to helping the child develop insight into his behaviors and to motivational interviews to help the child start on the path to recovery. It is also a time to adjust to living away from home, which some children do quickly and others more slowly. I was touched when Dr. Eken said that the children already in residence are very welcoming when new children arrive. The children know it's hard to live away from home. They try to help their new peers feel comfortable and safe while making the transition.

Dr. Eken pointed out that the availability of an inpatient unit at Rogers is also helpful. If a child should rapidly decompensate, a transfer there for stabilization is an option and she is able to follow her patient in that setting. In most residential programs, the child would have to be transferred to a completely different facility with new doctors. This raises an important question for you to ask the residential program you are considering: what will they do if your child suddenly falls apart?

Children in the residential program at Rogers receive classroom time with a certified teacher Monday through Friday of each week. Children in the Child Center receive two hours of instruction per day. The older children in the Adolescent Center receive one and a half hours per day. The teachers at Rogers communicate with the teachers at the child's home school to coordinate regarding areas of instruction. The goal is for the child to be academically on track when she returns home.

Out of curiosity, I asked Dr. Eken how OCD most often presents in her very young patients. She said, "Contamination and separation anxiety." She often finds a strong family history, a parent with OCD. In those cases, the parent is asked to pursue his or her own treatment as a model for the child. She did see one unusual case where a daughter was apparently mimicking her mother's OCD behaviors, but did not appear to have OCD herself.

Sometimes, the child arrives with a PANDAS diagnosis warranting a careful review of the blood work. Dr. Eken will review the records and run blood work to rule out the presence of an infection on all her patients. If she finds strep, her antibiotic of choice is Augmentin XR. She believes the clavulanic acid in the Augmentin may affect glutamate in the brain, which is a neurotransmitter involved in learning and memory.

If your child needs intensive help and you are exploring IOP as an alternative to a residential program, keep in mind that it requires a great deal of dedication and commitment from you and your child to succeed without the 24/7 oversight of trained professionals. In addition, the responsibility for schoolwork will fall on the parents' shoulders. For that reason, out-of-state IOPs are the most popular during the child's summer break from school.

SUMMING IT UP

There are a wide variety of residential programs throughout each state and specialized programs in only a few states. If your PANDAS child must enter a residential program, it will be because he needs a higher level of care than you can provide at home. Before placing your child, become fully familiar with the program and what it has to offer. It will not be productive for your child to end up living in a situation where those in charge do not accept the fact that behavioral disorders can be caused by an infection. Meet with those in charge, observe what is happening in the residence, find out about the other residents so you understand the profile of the program, familiarize yourself with the program's orientation, and understand the process for returning your child home. If your child is safe at home, but needs a more intensive CBT program than can be offered on an outpatient basis, consider the program offered at Rogers Memorial Hospital.

BIG IDEAS FROM CHAPTER FOURTEEN

❏ If residential care becomes necessary, you must do your homework before choosing a program.
❏ Visit and observe the program.
❏ Meet with the program director.
❏ Ask as many questions as you need to thoroughly understand the program.
❏ Review the program offered by Rogers Memorial Hospital and use it as a benchmark.
❏ Trust your instinct on whether a particular program is a good fit for you and your child.

Research And Resistance

15

Dear Beth,
Why does it take so long to figure this out and to convince doctors? I
keep trying to find a doctor to believe me and help my son. They all
say there's no reason to believe it exists or that antibiotics help. Will
this ever change?
Waiting Hopelessly

Dear Waiting,
It will change...but medicine moves at a snail's pace.
Beth

Hospitals, doctors, and medicine in general can be among the most frustrating or rewarding experiences in life depending upon the nature of the problem and quality of care. Where you go and who you see are crucial decisions. In the past, only doctors and other medical professionals were up to date about medicine; that is no longer true thanks to the Internet. It empowers us in many areas of life, and that includes health. The great secrets of medicine are not so mysterious after all and much of it is very straightforward. If you hear from a physician to "stay off the Internet" about PANDAS, you should take that as a sign to find a new doctor. Part of your job as a parent is to have as much information as possible. You won't change the closed mind of a doctor who has decided "there's no such thing as PANDAS," but knowledge is power.

Few among us are research scientists, so I collaborated with a number of them to bring you an understandable presentation of what they've been up to. By the time you read this even more studies may be available because research is always evolving, but here are some current highlights. Keep in mind that there are no PANS studies at present, just a reasonable hypothesis. Once upon a time though, PANDAS was merely a hypothesis, too.

By reading this chapter you will understand the broad strokes of reported research as well as be prepared for the nonbelievers you will encounter along the way. This chapter does not claim to cover all that is going on in the world of research or every theory about what may be involved in this disorder. I'm not a scientist, and I don't pretend to be one. If you are a researcher or consider yourself to be one, chances are you will want to do your own in-depth exploring.

Research

Thomas Insel, MD, director of the National Institute of Mental Health, wrote eloquently about the "controversy" over PANDAS/PANS in his Director's Blog of March 26, 2012, and drew a number of parallels to other challenges in mental health medicine. He explained that in the early 1900s many patients in mental asylums were diagnosed with "paresis," a form of psychosis with delusions, hallucinations, and memory problems attributed to a "general constitutional weakness." By 1917, however, the cause was identified as syphilis. Neuro-syphilis was effectively eliminated with the widespread availability of antibiotics in the late 1940s. He also blogged that in the 1970s peptic stomach ulcers (which you earlier read about in chapter 12, "Supports and Conflict"), were the prototype of a "biopsychosocial" disorder. Stress and Type A personalities were blamed as the cause, until 2005 when Barry Marshall, MD, and Robin Warren, MD, won the Nobel Prize in medicine for curing the ulcers with antibiotics.

What the doctor says:

"The idea that mental or behavioral disorders could be due to infection is not new, but remains surprisingly difficult to accept."

Thomas Insel, MD
National Institute of Mental Health
Director's Blog, March 26, 2012

Twenty to thirty years is not an abnormal timeframe for changes in medicine.

The Groundbreaker. Susan Swedo, MD, led the NIMH team that identified the bacterial link to obsessive-compulsive disorder in the late 1990s. Since then, hundreds of studies have been reported about PANDAS and related conditions, yet the nonbelievers persist. It's not particularly comforting, but the only conclusion to be drawn from the reluctance of the larger medical community to adapt to change is that such resistance is consistent with the history of medicine. We might hope things would be different in the new millennium, but they're not. The very vocal nonbelievers of PANDAS are doing nothing more than following in the footsteps of other misguided naysayers who preceded them. The research is there to be read; they are not interested. Parents, however, are forever grateful to the scientists and researchers who persist even as the nonbelievers try to shut them down.

Columbia Changes the Game. One of the most compelling pieces of research remains a mouse study that was published in August of 2009. In everyday language, it changed the game. A team of researchers led by Mady Hornig, MD, associate professor of epidemiology at Columbia University's Mailman School of Public Health, used a mouse model to demonstrate that strep antibodies produced obsessive-compulsive behaviors. Researchers infected one group of mice with strep bacteria. The mice produced antibodies to the infection and developed compulsive behaviors. Strep antibodies were then extracted from that first group of mice and introduced into a second group. The second group of mice then exhibited compulsive behaviors although they had never been exposed to the bacteria itself. The sudden presence of compulsive behaviors in the second group of mice indicated that strep antibodies were the cause. An example of compulsive behavior in mice is grooming themselves to the point that they strip off their fur.

FACT: When strep antibodies were extracted from mice engaged in compulsive behaviors and injected into a second group of mice, the second group exhibited the same behaviors.

Piercing the Blood-Brain Barrier. The blood-brain barrier (BBB), which normally protects the brain, was circumvented by Dr. Hornig and other researchers in earlier studies by direct injection of strep antibodies into the brain or by temporarily opening the BBB to allow entry of the antibodies. Thus, equally compelling is a 2012 paper by Danhui Zhang, PhD, and colleagues reporting that a single injection of strep antibodies into mice in the fatty layer of tissue between their skin and muscle (a subcutaneous injection) quickly induced stereotypical OCD behaviors such as head bobbing and intense self-grooming. The injection of control antibodies (those not for strep) did not have these effects. Importantly, the strep antibodies also stimulated activation of certain genes in brain areas relevant for these behaviors, and these antibodies were also found in the same brain areas. These results strongly support the hypothesis that strep infections cause the production of antibodies that can cross react with the brain, and directly alter neuronal activity and the animal's behavior. It was surprising that, in this study, no effort was made to disrupt (open) the BBB and yet the antibodies were able to enter the brain. By way of explanation, the authors suggested that the strain of mice they used is particularly susceptible to stress, and the mice were stressed by the injection and by the subsequent behavioral testing. Prior animal work showed that stress can temporarily open the BBB. This raises the possibility that stress could also be relevant in infection induction of the human conditions noted above.

> **FACT:** *Stress can temporarily open the blood-brain barrier.*

> 👉 *You must do everything you can to reduce your child's anxiety. Repeatedly reassure him that all will be well and never let him know when you are scared.*

The impact of stress. The "take away lesson" for parents from Dr. Zhang's research is that stress is one of your PANDAS child's worst enemies. For that reason alone, you must do all you can to reduce your child's anxiety by assuring her that all will be well. Those of you who have read *Saving Sammy* will remember the occasion when Sammy's compulsions and vocal tics reappeared upon returning from a trip to Florida. "It's back," he'd said to me with eyes full of fear. I was scared, too, but instinctively I comforted him. I said the tics were probably due to the weather change and that they would subside. The tics had grown steadily worse until that conversation, then they began to lessen within hours. I always thought his improvement had as much to do with my calm reassurance as adjusting to the colder weather, but why had remained a mystery. Because of Dr. Zhang's paper, I now understand that by telling Sammy that all would be well, thus reducing his stress level, I probably helped his BBB to close. This may also explain the anecdotal observations made by so many other parents that stress is a major factor in behavioral exacerbations. It is probably causing the BBB to open, thus permitting antibodies to cross into the brain.

Why mice? When Dr. Hornig's study was released, I was pleased it was so well received, but personally confused. Why was a mouse study considered pivotal instead of the case of a human boy named Sammy? What I learned about the beauty of laboratory mice is that they are, well, mice, with virtually no presenting variables. They do not attend school, have difficult peer relations, or otherwise engage in social situations that may cause emotional reactions and lead to disruptive behavior. Their parents do not divorce or move them about to different homes. In short, there was simply no reason for the second group of mice to begin engaging in compulsive behaviors other than the sudden introduction of strep antibodies. I also learned that because mice and humans share 95 percent of their genes, mice are an effective and efficient model for human disease. Demonstrating the link between the immune systems and the brains of mice supports the same connection in humans. Most important, there is more research flexibility with mice. Thankfully, strep antibodies will not be extracted from one group of children with OCD and then injected into a control group of children to see if symptoms develop.

The Immuno-Brain Link. The connection between the brain and the immune system is thoroughly explored by Paul H. Patterson, PhD in his book *Infectious Behavior*. Dr. Patterson, a developmental neurobiologist, is a professor at the California Institute of Technology and a research professor at the University of Southern

FACT:
Research indicates that the mother's inflammatory response during pregnancy is critical for altering fetal brain development.

California's Keck School of Medicine. He presents a powerful body of research demonstrating that across a range of mental health disorders the common thread is abnormalities in the immune system either in the mother, the patient, or both. He summarizes work showing that maternal infection, particularly during the first six months of pregnancy, increases the risk of schizophrenia in the offspring by as much as three- to sevenfold. He further reports that if a woman has a history of asthma or allergy, or an autoimmune disease such as rheumatoid arthritis or celiac disease, it approximately doubles the likelihood that her child will have autism or an autism spectrum disorder. The conclusion he draws is that the mother's inflammatory response is critical for altering fetal brain development.

Dr. Patterson's reports are confirmed by research conducted by Tanya K. Murphy, MD, who holds the Rothman Endowed Chair of Developmental Pediatrics in the Departments of Pediatrics and Psychiatry at the University of South Florida. The medical histories of the biological mothers of 107 children with OCD and/or tics were reviewed for the study. In December of 2010, the results were published. Autoimmune disorders were reported in 17.8 percent of study mothers compared with the general prevalence among women across the United States (approximately 5 percent). Further, study mothers were more likely to report having an autoimmune disease if their children were considered "likely PANDAS" cases versus "unlikely PANDAS" cases.

Making sure the immune system is healthy may offer great help to the brain; the relationship between the two is indisputable.

Given the breath of research linking the immune system to brain disorders, it remains puzzling why so many in the medical community are still forcing doctors and advocates to push that bolder uphill.

Why Brain Circuits Fail. Madeleine Cunningham, PhD, is a professor at the University of Oklahoma Health Sciences Center. Her lab has investigated molecular mimicry, autoimmunity, and infection in inflammatory heart disease with a focus on strep for the past thirty years. Molecular mimicry is when the immune system misfires and makes antibodies to a foreign bacterial or virus (molecule) that also cross-reacts with (or mistakenly attack) a similar molecule, one that is not the pathogen. Dr. Cunningham's lab identified the antibody-induced cell signaling that causes the chorea movements present in Sydenham's chorea, the movement disorder associated with rheumatic fever.

FACT: *Research has identified that strep antibodies stimulate brain proteins and change the way that brain cells send signals.*

Dr. Cunningham wondered if she could identify the cell signaling that causes the behaviors in PANDAS children, so she began to study the blood of children diagnosed with PANDAS. One of the brain proteins involved in antibody-induced cell signaling is CaM kinase II. By placing strep antibodies obtained from the blood of PANDAS patients in a culture with a human neuronal (brain) cell line, Dr. Cunningham's study group observed that CaM kinase II was stimulated. When the chemical balance in the brain changes, behavior is affected. By identifying that strep antibodies are stimulating CaM kinase II, thus changing the way brain cells send signals, researchers may now understand why the PANDAS children's behaviors are abnormal. Dr. Cunningham's first PANDAS study was reported in the *Journal of Neuroimmunology* in 2006. In 2013, Dr. Cunningham co-founded Moleculera Labs, which offers a blood panel that assesses whether PANDAS/PANS is highly likely, likely, or not likely. Information about the Cunningham Panel can be found on the lab's website at www.moleculera.com.

Why Does Augmentin Work So Well? The question that personally nags me was prompted by my own experience with Sammy and confirmed by the clinical observations of so many doctors and e-mails from parents. Why does Augmentin consistently produce the best antibiotic response? Augmentin has two components: amoxicillin (a penicillin-based medication) and clavulanic acid. Most children respond to Augmentin far better than amoxicillin or penicillin. Logically, it must be something about the clavulanic acid. Kevin Price,

MD, the open-minded surgeon, wondered if clavulanic acid might have an anti-inflammatory effect. He suggested that measuring ESR (erythrocyte sedimentation rate) or CRP (C-reactive protein) levels checked after administration of clavulanic acid alone might offer a clue. ESR and CRP are measures of inflammation that can be taken through blood. Dr. Patterson at Caltech thought this was an interesting idea and is exploring this possibility. If his lab at Caltech ultimately unlocks the key about clavulanic acid, the implications will extend far beyond PANDAS and may potentially impact treatments for other disorders such as Parkinson's, Alzheimer's, Lupus, and Lyme.

Forging Forward. Current and pending research offers great promise. Dr. Susan Swedo of the NIMH and Dr. James Lechtman of Yale spearheaded research launched in early 2011 designed to study whether IV Ig might be an effective treatment for PANDAS children. Aside from the medical implications, if these doctors can demonstrate its efficacy, the study may help parents who are fighting insurance carriers for coverage of this treatment. During that same year, Eric Storch, PhD, at the University of South Florida reported that D-Cycloserine, an "old" antibiotic used to treat tuberculosis, had a positive effect on the learning curve of patients engaged in cognitive behavioral therapy. This antibiotic does not address the underlying infection, but rather improves the patient's ability to modify his behaviors. Another piece of interesting research about how best to treat "persisters" was reported in *Nature* in the spring of 2011 and summarized by *Discover* magazine. Persisters are the bacteria that evade antibiotics by essentially going dormant only to flare up again once the danger has passed. This sounds remarkably similar to what PANDAS children experience with recurring infections. Author James Collins said the goal of researching the persisters was essentially how to "get them up off the ground so we can punch them and knock them out." The paper reported that when antibiotics were combined directly with sugar and placed in a petrie dish, over 99 percent of bacterial persisters were killed. The persisters simply could not resist the sugar. If you think of bacteria as fish, then sugar is the worm and the antibiotic is the hook. In 2012, Tanya Murphy, MD launched a research study designed to track the response of PANDAS children to azithromycin. Daniel Geller, MD is currently exploring the possibility of an Augmentin study.

What's Left? We need to understand exactly what happens in the body and brain to produce a behavioral disorder. After endless meetings, discussions, conferences, and telephone calls, my guess is that it's the neurobiologists who will someday answer that question. Only with that answer in place, will targeted treatment be developed with certainty. In the meantime though, we need doctors to treat our children based on the experience of practitioners who know what works. Doctors don't always know exactly why a particular medication works, but they prescribe it because it produces the desired result. Dr. Nicolaides told me years ago when Sammy was first sick that she knew Augmentin was the antibiotic that produced the best result for PANDAS children, she just didn't know why. Careful, capable, intelligent doctors who will responsibly treat a patient with what works, even when they cannot explain exactly why, are the kind of doctors that you need to find for your PANDAS child.

In the future, all of us may be able to look back and understand why a particular medication worked; but your child needs help now, long before we have those answers.

What the doctor says:

"Even in the early 1990s, a syphilis screen was a routine step in psychiatry for patients with psychiatric symptoms. I don't know how much syphilis is around today, but the point is that it was still in our repertoire to look for physical causes. No psychiatry does that anymore."

Tanya Murphy, MD

Resistance

Dear Beth,

What if the school nurse, et al do not believe in PANDAS? Think it's "tsk tsk... controversial" and you are a parent in denial because your child has Tourette's, etc.? This is what I'm wondering. We start a new school this week. The old one was in the dark about it — cuz so were we. But now we know better and are trying to figure out how to bring them along.

Dealing with the Dark Ages

> *Dear Dealing,*
>
> *I'd tell them they're working from old information. Mention there are hundreds of studies that verify PANDAS and direct them to the NIMH webpage. Have them take a look at the PANDAS information on the website for the International OCD Foundation, including the PSA from Harvard's Dr. Michael Jenike. Remind them about syphilis, stomach ulcers, and childbed fever. Mention that "controversial" is a word that is used to squelch medicine—not advance it. Then I'd hand them a copy of this book along with Saving Sammy.*
>
> *Beth*

Each way you turn you may face obstacles. Overcoming some of these obstacles is covered in chapter 12, "Supports and Conflict." Others might appear insurmountable, but understanding what you are up against will help. One may be obtaining insurance coverage. Another may be the troublesome nonbelievers, who play by their own set of rules.

The Health Insurance Web. It's tough enough to find a willing provider and get your child properly diagnosed, but the hurdles posed by health insurance companies may be equally challenging. Logically, health insurers should be one of the biggest advocates for appropriate diagnosis and treatment of PANDAS. After all, the cost of treatment with antibiotics, an infusion with IV Ig, cognitive behavioral therapy sessions, and even a short stay in a residential program cannot compare with the cost of long-term psychiatric illness both to insurers and to society as a whole. Yet, mental health coverage has long been considered the black sheep of the family and health insurance companies typically limit non-prescription aspects of mental health benefits both by dollar amount and number of visits. And although lifelong psychotropic medication prescribed for psychosis will be routinely covered, insurers will sometimes balk at long-term antibiotic coverage or coverage with certain antibiotics. At least two carriers—United Healthcare and Harvard Pilgrim—have excluded coverage for IV Ig in PANDAS children. Blue Cross/Blue Shield seems to be moving in that direction as well.

I wish I had a good explanation for what feels like uninformed and arbitrary decision-making.

Coverage often depends on how the insurer is structured. If

one insurer internally covers both the physical and mental health pieces, they may be more likely to recognize that in the long run, by addressing mental health ailments appropriately, they will be saving physical health expenditures. Often though, the mental health benefit is farmed out to a different carrier so the "cost benefit" analysis falls on deaf ears. As far as residential coverage, there is no double blind placebo study showing that CBT works. As a result, stays in residential programs are often denied. The standard for inpatient treatment is often whether the patient is a risk to himself or others. A suicidal patient will be admitted to the hospital, but once the crisis is passed he must be quickly sent home. Moreover, mental health coverage decisions are often subject to "review" by physicians who function as independent contractors. If they say "yes" too often, they'll lose their contracts. They risk nothing by saying "no" when a different answer might have saved a life.

If you are in the process of buying health insurance, and PANDAS is an issue for your child, you need to ask a lot of questions. What is the mental health benefit? What will happen if my child is hospitalized for a mental health disorder? Is IV Ig excluded? Does the insurance company farm the mental health benefit out to a third party "reinsurer?" If you are already in a situation with an insurer who is denying coverage, keep in mind that extraordinary advocacy may sometimes help. If your child needs a residential program to overcome obsessive-compulsive behaviors, remember that this is one area of mental health where clear tools and treatment parameters can help your child. It will require great personal strength and advocacy to stand up to an insurance company. If you need help, this may be a time when you need to consider hiring an attorney.

Insurance implications are one of the reasons why there are a limited number of child psychiatrists. Doctors who very much want to treat children must pause to consider the financial realities. Medical students, like lawyers, can choose to practice their skills in any one of a number of different areas. When faced with huge medical school loans and families to support, the financial reality of a particular area of practice is a valid consideration. When a psychiatrist spends an hour with a child, insurance reimbursement for services will often be in the area of $110. If an orthopedic surgeon spends fifteen minutes with a patient and orders an MRI, the reimbursement will often be $250. Given the dollars involved, is it any wonder why it's easier to find an orthopedic surgeon than a child psychiatrist? It certainly explains why many PANDAS doctors are private pay. I don't fault the doctors. I fault the fact that mental and physical health should be—but are not—on equal footing. Given that suicide is the third leading cause of death among teenagers, developing an effective mental health system with adequate providers should be a national priority.

Mental health policy and perspective need to change. Various reports issued by the Surgeon General's office and the National Health Policy Forum estimate that about 20 percent of children in the United States have mental health disorders ranging from mild to severe. Less than half of these children receive treatment. One in twenty, or about 5 percent of all children, have serious dysfunction. Cancer, by comparison, is estimated to afflict approximately 2 percent of all children. Why then does mental health remain relegated to second-class status? Part of the problem is that our society as a whole does not think mental illness is "real." Think of the struggle you have faced in having PANDAS accepted as a viable disorder even among your immediate circle of acquaintances.

Nonbelievers. The question I am always asked when I give presentations is, "Why don't some doctors believe in PANDAS?" I always struggle to find the answer. One clear reason is that not all doctors are created equal. It seems obvious in retrospect. Yet, before Sammy was sick, I had put all doctors on the same pedestal and placed it so high that I had to stand on my tiptoes and squint to see it. The fact is that there are wide variations among doctors, just as in any profession. Some are better, smarter, more talented, and more open-minded than others.

Then there is the nature of medicine itself, with its concerning history of arrogance. Once medicine takes a position, it stays there for a very long time. Medicine boasts a long, unfortunate history of nonbelievers proven wrong, and the examples are poignant: childbed fever, stomach ulcers, and Freud's misguided theories about behaviors. These all took scores of years to overcome. In short, the medical community is comfortable with what it knows, and sometimes has to be dragged kicking and screaming out of its comfort zone. The conservative approach may lead to careful medicine but, unfortunately, a standard that rigid can also bring progress to a grinding halt. It can cause medical inertia. If a child is transformed from a normal, healthy little guy into an unrecognizable version of his former self, logic dictates that introducing a course of antibiotics to see if it might help makes sense. Medical inertia dictates waiting for more research studies before taking that logical step.

Research studies—the security blanket of medicine—take years to develop, fund, and then eventually publish. Once published, doctors then like to see the study results replicated—multiple times. Again patients wait, even though they've already been waiting a very long time. Medical research generally confirms years of prior clinical observations. So for medicine to progress, brave doctors need to follow their clinical instincts and treat, which—when it happens enough—eventually and slowly leads to research studies. Sometimes doctors are brave enough; others are not. "I don't believe in it," is a catchall phrase that is often used as an excuse to do nothing.

Then there are the politics and rivalries of medicine. Even in medical school, there are hierarchies and territorial aspects to the different specialties. Pediatricians, the doctors on whom parents most often rely, are not considered to be at the top. Given that the pediatrician is the doctor your child will see the most until she is eighteen, and may see more regularly than any other doctor during her lifetime, who could be more important? Insurance reimbursement rates reflect society's perception of the value of a doctor's particular specialty. Children are not as important as they should be so reimbursements are low. Lack of mental health is someone else's fault or problem.

Then, of course, one cannot overlook gender. The leading nonbelievers are primarily men. The leading PANDAS researchers are primarily women. But the publication of *Saving Sammy* in 2009 changed the dynamics, and I think the odds look quite good. Thousands of parents with sick children have stepped forward onto the medical landscape and taken hold of this disorder. A few doctors may be able to intimidate a few other doctors, but not thousands of determined parents.

Like a bad penny though, the nonbelievers keep turning up, stuck on their old-school views. In January 2012, under the memorable caption "Medical Progress," five nonbelieving doctors published "Moving from PANDAS to CANS." The paper advocated that the diagnosis of PANDAS be eliminated. In short, that an entire area of medicine be shut down. The article ran in the *Journal of Pediatrics* and put forth the position that children should not be treated with antibiotics for acute onset of tics, OCD, and other neuropsychiatric symptoms. In making their points, they failed to mention the vast body of Dr. Tanya Murphy's research (more than 140 authored papers) supporting the link between strep and obsessive-compulsive disorder. They also failed to mention their conflicts of interests, which were then printed in the journal's next issue.

The authors advocated for prescribing psychotropic medication and administering invasive procedures to your children. Demonstrating their disconnection from reality, they raised questions such as whether behaviors could be considered "immediate onset," if it took as much as ten days for a child to go from baseline to completely dysfunctional. They're apparently clueless that it really doesn't matter if it takes one day, one week, or one month for sweet, healthy, normal children to become unrecognizable. The point is that the child you loved and nurtured is suddenly gone. Last week she was humming tunes while she painted pictures of birds and flowers. This week she's slamming her head into the wall. One truly has to wonder what would motivate doctors to recommend prescribing psychotropic medication that alters the brain's chemistry and putting a child through a battery of painful, expensive testing rather than trying a noninvasive, simple, relatively inexpensive course of antibiotics.

SUMMING IT UP

The future is bright. No area of medicine has come so far, so fast, as has PANDAS and that is due to the full-court press of parents following the publication of *Saving Sammy* in 2009. At that time, research had basically come to a standstill. There were only a handful of doctors treating PANDAS and no support groups existed. The International OCD Foundation did not support the diagnosis and the NIMH web page was woefully out of date. All that has changed because of parents. We have shared our stories, spoken our truth, and loudly demanded that the infectious basis for our children's behaviors be appropriately addressed. The national news media has helped focus the public's attention on this formerly obscure disorder. Research has been reinvigorated. And for the first time ever, in October of 2013, both the American Academy of Pediatrics (AAP) and the American Academy of Child and Adolescent Psychiatry (AACAP) featured

PANDAS presentations at their annual conferences. Dr. Susan Swedo, Dr. Tanya Murphy, and Dr. Madeleine Cunningham were all presenters.

Ultimately, the controversy will be laid to rest, and infections will routinely be considered when children present with behavioral disorders. Years from now, parents will take for granted that infections cause mental illness the way we take for granted that doctors should scrub between patients, that infections can cause stomach ulcers, and that syphilis attacks the brain. When our children are parents, they will look back and wonder why there was ever an issue; the same way we look back and wonder why women were ever precluded from voting, becoming doctors, or practicing law.

The problem is that day will not come soon enough.

BIG IDEAS FROM CHAPTER FIFTEEN

- ❏ Medicine moves at the opposite speed of a cheetah.
- ❏ The Internet is your friend.
- ❏ Mice are your friends, too, and share 95 percent of their genes with you.
- ❏ Mice can develop compulsive behaviors from strep antibodies.
- ❏ Stress can temporarily open the blood-brain barrier.
- ❏ The link between the brain and the immune system has been repeatedly reported in studies.
- ❏ When there are strep antibodies in the brain, they change the way that brain cells send signals.
- ❏ There is a vast body of research supporting PANDAS.
- ❏ Insurance companies are often not your friend.
- ❏ Not all doctors are created equal.
- ❏ The nonbelievers publish papers that fail to distinguish conflicting research and fail to disclose their conflicts of interest.
- ❏ The parents are winning.

VI WHEN IT'S OVER

The Gift of Recovery

16

Dear Beth,

I'm sure you have received tons of letters thanking you for all you have done for so many. Here's one more. My daughter was a very sick little girl one year ago. Her tics and OCD consumed her days. She was completely nonfunctional. She did not smile, laugh, talk, or leave our house. She was always in distress and cried for hours especially at night. I took her to Cincinnati Children's Hospital where they diagnosed her with OCD. She was put on antidepressants, antipsychotics, and anti-seizure medication. She also did CBT for nine months. None of it worked. My sister-in-law saw your story and shared it with me. Sammy's story seemed an awful lot like what we were going through. Not surprising I couldn't get one doctor to buy into it. I finally took her to see Sammy's doctor, Catherine Nicolaides, MD. We met with her seven months ago, four days after Missy's tenth birthday. What a birthday present that turned out to be! Missy is back to being the happy, sweet, funny girl she always was. Life is normal, boring in the very best possible way! Thank you seems so insignificant to say, when your story and your work gave my daughter and our family our lives back. I hope you are repaid and rewarded everyday for your dedication to this disease. If there is anything I can ever do to help, please let me know. You are our hero!

Missy's Mom

Despite the passage of years, there are still times when what happened to us leaves me breathless and wondering how we managed to pull through. It most often catches me when I read a passage from *Saving Sammy* at a presentation and find myself fighting hard to hold back tears. It happens when I counsel one of you by telephone. I hear the fear and desperation in your voice, and I remember. Whenever it happens, the hopelessness of those days rushes back and engulfs me. I remember the darkness of a hole so deep that I thought we'd never climb out. I remember Sammy too ill to eat or step outside. Mostly I remember the agony: my son buried under the cushions of our couch for months, my heart in tatters on the floor, doctors who left me without hope, who said I was wrong, and did so without a shred of understanding about what our lives had become. But I also remember the love of my family and friends who supported me, unearthing the NIMH research, a glimmer of hope when I e-mailed my early thoughts to Tanya Murphy, MD, and she sent back, "I could not agree more." The successful struggle to—finally—find the doctors who treated Sammy and believed recovery was possible. Then—at last—the miracle. First baby steps, then leaps and bounds, as Sammy regained his health. My home was filled with laughter and sibling squabbling again because as Sammy healed, so did we all.

Is there anything more precious than reclaiming a life?

I distinctly recall a particular moment from the summer of Sammy's recovery. He was getting ready to head back to school that fall for the first time in two years. With tutoring, he was finishing up the curriculum from the year before, and he needed a book. I slid the van into a parking space in front of our red-brick local library. I was about to turn the van off and hop out to walk in with him when he said, "I can go in myself, Mom." I turned, studied his determined face, and nodded to him, "Okay, love. I'll run a few errands, and then I'll come back." As I watched him walk up the path, climb the stairs, and open the big green door to the library, I wondered: How many moms take a simple moment like this for granted? I promised myself that I never would. I've thanked God for every one of those moments: heading off to high school, flying off to college, and—next thing I knew—joining me on the *Today Show* and joking with Matt Lauer.

> *Dear Beth,*
> *When I reached out to you last month I was at the end of my rope. Your response and phone call came at just the right moment and was nothing short of a miracle. We asked the doctor to run all the tests that you suggested. They did even though I don't think they expected much to come of it. Those test results have changed the course of how doctors*

*are approaching diagnosis and treatment. After years of despair,
there is hope. We can never thank you enough.*
   Very Grateful Mom

I particularly recall one day in Los Angeles while Sammy and I were waiting to go on *The Doctors*. We were backstage in the dressing room, busily running through the format for the show with the producer and meeting some of the other guests. The producer, needing to attend to additional details, handed us some forms to sign and said she'd be back in a few minutes. I breezed through my forms and looked up to see Sammy casually leaning on a counter, relaxed and signing his paperwork.

"Sammy," I said, "look here." He turned those deeply intelligent brown eyes toward me. I used my phone to snap the photo that was later posted on my Facebook fan page. This remarkable young man, my precious son, was sharing his life again in the interest of healing so many others. I'd have given my own life for him, for any one of my children, if God would grant them health. God gave him back to me and, in so doing, granted me my life back, too. I believe this all happened because we were meant to fulfill a greater purpose. Sammy's generosity in allowing me to tell his story has significantly changed the face of mental illness for children, and set my own life on a path I never imagined. This book is part of that trajectory.

Dear Beth,
*Please keep doing what you do. Every time I hit a brick wall, you
are there to pick up the pieces. Life is messy and crazy, but everything
falls back into place when I see an interview of yours or read a letter
you send us parents. I know your goal is to reach out and help us get
there! I am getting there with your help...you are like our guiding
angel. Thank you.*
   Parent of Another Child Who Caught OCD

After all the hard work, the articles, appearances, conferences, and tireless advocacy, it is frustrating that so many of you still found out about PANDAS by happenstance. I have heard almost every variation. Someone handed you this book because they heard about what was going on with your child. A relative happened to see us on television, or hear a radio broadcast. Your school nurse mentioned that she had heard something about this. You stumbled across *Saving Sammy* in the library. Your child's diagnosis didn't add up, so you did your own research and found me through the Internet. You are friends with someone, who has a friend in another state, whose child came down with PANDAS. Thumbing through a magazine at the child psychiatrist's office, you came across an article and insisted your child be tested for strep. What I almost never hear is, "My doctor told me." What I regularly hear is, "My doctor doesn't believe in it."

I know you are facing a long road ahead and seemingly insurmountable odds, but don't give up. You can do it. Find the courage buried deep within you. Do for your child what you might not have the strength to do for yourself. Model for them what it's like to fight as a parent. Stick up for yourself when others are dismissive. Fire the doctors who roll their eyes. Don't be sidetracked by people who stand in your way. Hold determinedly to the vision of your child as healthy and well, don't be dissuaded, and never let that vision go. When you have finished fighting tooth and nail to get your child the help he needs, and he finally stands before you one day well, smiling, and looking forward to the life you've given back to him, there will be no greater gift. Accept that gift and share it. Tell everyone you know about PANDAS: talk to other parents, teachers, and to school nurses, mention it in grocery store lines, accost people in elevators, bring it up at parent meetings. Discuss it at backyard barbecues and while your children play soccer. Ask your mother to tell her friends. Give doctors this book. There isn't time to wait for the greater medical community to come to the realization that a simple infection can cause mental illness. We have to push it, every day.

Then please do one more thing for me: wrap your child in your arms and tell your sweet bundle of love that you're passing along a big hug from me—because you are not alone.

Beth
info@savingsammy.net

Hello!

My name is Samantha. I'm from New Jersey, and I'm fourteen years old. Ever since I was twelve years old, I've had what they thought was psychological. I've been on every medication—Prozac, Paxil, Adderall, Vyvanse, Kapvay, Klonopin, Xanax, Lorazepam, Zoloft, Depakote, Risperidone, Effexor—a whole cocktail of medications. For the last few years, I've been hopping medications and doctors. In February of this year, I started to be homeschooled because of panic attacks. In March, I was admitted into a psychiatric hospital. My symptoms were panic attacks, depression, severe anxiety, OCD, and tics. Not as severe as your son. The panic attacks were the worst; they lasted hours of screaming, crying, shaking, and violence toward myself and my surroundings. In May, my mom found out about PANDAS. We went to Dr. Rosario Trifiletti (I'm not sure how you spell his name) in New Jersey. He diagnosed me with PANDAS. I had a blood test. I was carrying strep, mono, walking pneumonia, a pneumococcal infection, and I was missing vital vitamins and proteins in my blood. I was taken off everything but Klonopin, and I had Xanax for emergencies. I was put on Amoxicillin for ten days and supplements. Everything but my anxiety disappeared. About a week after finishing the antibiotic, my neck and jaw tics came back. I had more panic attacks. I started a round of Augmentin XR, 1,000mg. Ever since then, my anxiety has been suppressed, but it's still there. My tics only arise out of stress. My iron level doubled and I am continuing to take my supplements. I finished the Klonopin. Recently, I had a scare. I had symptoms of strep. My throat culture was negative, and the symptoms faded. I have a few tics and anxiety, but I think it's just from the stress of the new school year.

Recently, both my mother and I have read *Saving Sammy*. Reading it gave me so much hope. I've always felt so alone in this. I knew there were other kids out there, but I haven't heard of anyone before I read your book.

Thank you for getting Sammy's story out. I'm so thankful for you.

Sincerely,
Samantha, Age 14

Viewpoints: Treating Physicians

Hello Beth,

Thank you for your website and your strength to share your story. Three weeks ago after a minor cold and cough, my 4 year old daughter began refusing to wear clothes because they are dirty. She will not sit and is constantly wiping the house or herself. Prior to this, she was a fun-loving little, blue-eyed girl with ringlet curls. My heart is breaking. She tested positive for strep three days ago and has started Augmentin and steroids. Do you have a physician who specializes in PANDAS? We can't find anyone, and I will fly to whomever you recommend.

Warmly,

Broken Hearted

The current list of treating physicians can always be found from the pull down menu of Other Resources on savingsammy. net. Unfortunately, there is limited availability. Therefore, what follows are the viewpoints of a number of physicians, who are recognized by other physicians and by caregivers as being skilled in treating PANDAS. Contact information for each of these doctors is provided at the end of this appendix. Some of the doctors confine their practice to treating patients; others are also on the forefront of research. I interviewed each of these doctors, either by telephone or in person, and then compiled the information. Each doctor was given the opportunity to review and approve my presentation of his or her perspective.

Because no treatment protocol is available to guide your own physician, perhaps he or she might read these viewpoints for guidance. Whether you are reading this chapter as a doctor or a caregiver, my hope is that you will find a treatment method or related information that is a good fit for you. As with the rest of the book, this section is not intended and should not be construed as medical advice. It merely provides the approaches of experienced doctors across the country as a starting point for discussing the types of intervention that may prove helpful. Although some of the doctors may describe the use of a particular psychotropic medication, this book does not discuss those medications themselves, as that would be a book in itself. For detailed information on different psychotropic medications, you might consider *Straight Talk about Psychiatric Medications for Kids* by Timothy E. Wilens, MD.

DAVID BAND, M.D.

David Band, M.D. is a psychiatrist with offices in Virginia and Maryland. He estimates that in the past ten years he has treated close to 100 patients with PANDAS.

When Dr. Band first started treating PANDAS patients, he looked for sudden onset of obsessive-compulsive symptoms or tics. Even with those symptoms, he did not treat it without elevated titers. Now his approach is very different. He will consider PANDAS if there is the sudden onset of any repetitive behaviors. For example, when someone comes in and states, "this started last Tuesday," he immediately thinks of PANDAS. He occasionally sees PANDAS present as panic, anxiety, ADHD, or any combination thereof without any significant OCD or tic symptoms. He also learned through experience that PANDAS can present as an extreme exacerbation of any of the previously mentioned symptoms. A complete absence of prior behaviors is not necessary for the diagnosis. There may be some minor behaviors in the background, perhaps even for years, which suddenly explode. It's as if someone abruptly turns up the volume to an excruciating level. When Dr. Band believes a child has PANDAS, he orders blood work, but often starts treatment before the results come back. Most of his PANDAS patients do have elevated titers, but his experience has shown that some children respond even without an elevated titer. Even if the titers are not elevated, Dr. Band is likely to continue treatment once it is started.

When he sees a patient who has experienced a gradual development of symptoms, and/or a moderate improvement or fluctuation of symptoms, Dr. Band is less likely to feel the patient has PANDAS. Nonetheless, he will sometimes order titer tests for these children as well because, while PANDAS is unlikely, it is not impossible. However, until proven differently, he believes the patient likely has Lyme when the presentation is joint pain combined with changes in mood, physical, and neurological state (depression, irritability, frustration, anger, rage, impatience, short-term memory difficulties, confusion, changes in ability to focus, fatigue, weakness, sedation, changes in pain perception and sensitivity to light and/or sound, changes in muscle strength and coordination with actual loss of muscle mass). "Not all Lyme patients have joint pain, though," added Dr. Band. "My daughter never had joint pain, but she has Lyme. We found out because after several visits to the pediatrician, I insisted that she get a Lyme titer."

Most of Dr. Band's PANDAS patients respond to antibiotics. His first choice is Augmentin, and he starts at a low dose. He prefers to start slowly because many patients have a hard time tolerating Augmentin as GI (gastrointestinal) symptoms can develop. He carefully monitors the patient's response and increases the dosage as needed. He does not use the Extended Release version of Augmentin initially because those pills are 1000 mg, and he prefers to have more flexibility starting at a lower dose given two to four times a day depending upon tolerability. If the patient cannot tolerate Augmentin, he may try amoxicillin instead, although a more probable choice is Omnicef. Omnicef is always his first choice for a patient allergic to penicillin (both Augmentin and amoxicillin are penicillin based). He usually prescribes pills, but occasionally a patient needs the liquid formulation.

When treatment begins with antibiotics, Dr. Band tries to avoid prescribing new or changing existing psychotropic medication. He only wants to change one thing at a time, so that he can obtain an accurate measure of the children's response to the antibiotics. He has noticed that patients tend to see him in clusters. He may go for months without a single PANDAS patient and then may see three patients within two weeks. Dr. Band does his best to educate the patients' pediatricians and primary care doctors about PANDAS by faxing them information about the disorder along with his treatment recommendations. Most are responsive, while others are not and sometimes challenge him about whether a strep infection can cause behavioral symptoms. "Remember back in medical school when we learned about St. Vitus's Dance (Sydenham's chorea)? " He'll remind them this is a movement disorder caused by strep. Periodically, he will send the physicians updates about the children's behaviors.

Diligently taking family and social histories are crucial parts of effective treatment for Dr. Band, so he asks a lot of questions. With enough persistence and patience, when he suspects PANDAS, he usually finds a strep infection lurking somewhere. It might be the patient, but sometimes it is another family member who was previously treated for a strep infection. He has also discovered the source to be a visiting relative, a family member of a friend, or another individual with whom the patient has had contact. The child might have been slightly ill at the time, but not sick enough to see the doctor.

Asking enough questions is what solved one of Dr. Band's most puzzling PANDAS cases. It involved a patient being treated with liquid Augmentin. She was doing quite well, but then her mother called to schedule an early appointment because the child's behaviors were returning. Two days before her appointment, she was suddenly doing better again. Dr. Band felt there had to be an explanation. By asking enough questions, he realized that the pharmacy had provided the girl with a month's worth of reconstituted liquid Augmentin. Liquid Augmentin is prepared or "reconstituted" by mixing the powdered medication with water. Each bottle is only at full strength for ten days. By the time 14 days have passed, the Augmentin has become as much as 60 percent less effective. The Augmentin simply stopped working because, in essence, the patient was taking less and less active medication over the last two weeks of her thirty-day prescription. The patient started a freshly reconstituted bottle just days before her appointment, which explained her recent improvement. By ensuring the girl always had fresh medicine (a newly reconstituted bottle of Augmentin every 10 days), she returned to the path of recovery.

Now, Dr. Band always alerts parents to the potential problem so they can make certain they receive their monthly medication in three bottles, only one of which is reconstituted at the time it is picked up at the pharmacy. Each of the others can easily be reconstituted by parents on the first day it is needed by simply adding the correct amount of water. If any medication remains after 10 days, parents should discard it in an environmentally safe manner and start the next bottle. Never pour medication down the drain or flush it down the toilet. This prevents it from entering the water system. Your pharmacist can provide you with information on proper ways to dispose of unused medications of all types. Many cities and towns have semi-annual collections of unused prescription medications for environmentally safe disposal.

Dr. Band is certified by the American Board of Psychiatry and Neurology in psychiatry.

ALI CARINE, D.O.

Ali Carine, D.O. is a pediatrician in Columbus, Ohio who integrates mainstream medicine with holistic, nutritional, and lifestyle approaches. She has been treating PANDAS patients since 2006 and estimates that she sees about 3-6 new PANDAS patients a week. As an integrative pediatrician, Dr. Carine considers all aspects of the child and his environment when she is the treating physician. This philosophy views illness as a combination of the infectious organism and the patient's response to that organism. In the case of PANDAS, if one approaches only the bacteria by using antibiotics, then the autoimmunity is allowed to continue. This makes the condition more difficult to control. Therefore, her approach is two fold: address the immune dysfunction and treat the infection. She believes this combination of treating the whole child has led to better control and less use of long-term antibiotics, even when she begins treatment years into the illness.

Because her practice includes primary care patients from birth and she takes insurance, she often sees children in the early stages of PANDAS. Their parents often bring them in for minor complaints of bedwetting, school anxiety, poor sleep, ADHD, or poor school performance. The parents are often surprised when she suggests blood work for ASO titers and Anti-DNase B, but these are very often positive. She finds it very rewarding to be able to find these cases early. If she sees a response to the antibiotics within a day or two then her instincts are confirmed, and she finds that most of the children she tests come back with elevated titers. However, Dr. Carine feels the key is not whether the titer is high, but rather if the child responds with improved behaviors after the antibiotics. The relative number of the titers does not always correlate with the severity of the disease, but children with very high titers, over 1000, do seem to require more antibiotics to treat. Her antibiotics of choice are Omnicef first and Zithromax second.

Dr. Carine feels that antibiotics alone make it difficult to control the disease. So she looks hard for other reasons for immune system dysfunction. Many children she sees are gluten intolerant. She said it is well known that gluten intolerance can trigger autoimmune disease. For that reason, she believes parents should seek genetic testing for celiac or consider a trial gluten-free diet to see if it helps. She also recommends other dietary changes and supplements to improve immune function. One of those supplements is Curcumin, the active ingredient in Turmeric, which is in the same family of spices as curry. This is known for a number of helpful qualities primarily related to decreasing autoimmune activity and neuro-regulatory effects. For an aggressive child, Dr. Carine recommends eliminating milk as well.

Dr. Carine has rarely had to prescribe more than five or six rounds of antibiotics in early stages of treatment, and all but a few of her cases have been contained. In Dr. Carine's experience, once a child has had a PANDAS episode then the symptoms will return when the child is put under stress: either fatigue, viral infections, or injuries. Parents should watch for returning symptoms and be quick to start antibiotics again. The cases she finds most difficult to contain are in autistic children or when the child continues to be exposed through other family members. She finds that if the parent returns the child to his previous diet, stops the supplements, in short fails to manage the condition on an ongoing basis, then PANDAS will return or perhaps another autoimmune dysfunction may develop.

"Even with chronic kids, if you treat them holistically, they need fewer antibiotics." Dr. Carine said. "I have only a handful that have needed long term antibiotics. I believe there are many kids whose parents think they don't have PANDAS because, 'they have been this way their whole life,' and no one ever checked. So, I see those kids too, and they are often positive, frequently dramatically so. It surprises me everyday how many positives I see."

Dr. Carine is certified by the American Osteopathic Board of Pediatrics, and by The American Osteopathic Board of Neuromusculoskeletal Medicine.

DANIEL A. GELLER, M.D.

Daniel Geller, M.D. is a child psychiatrist who founded and is the director of the Pediatric OCD and Tic Disorder Program at Massachusetts General Hospital. Dr. Geller has treated about 100 PANDAS patients beginning with my son Sammy. In addition to treating patients through Massachusetts General and in his private practice, Dr. Geller is one of the leading researchers in the country in pediatric OCD. "We don't really understand fully all the pathogens that can cause neuropsychiatric symptoms," he said. He believes that along with strep, other infections such as mycoplasma, Lyme, and perhaps some viruses may trigger post infectious autoimmune neurobehavioral disorders for example, PANS: Pediatric Acute-Onset Neuropsychiatric Syndrome. Most of the children Dr. Geller has treated recover, and he is looking for a complete resolution of all symptoms.

Dr. Geller finds that parents are bringing their children to him at an earlier stage in the disorder as awareness has grown. While Dr. Geller thinks the field is still in its infancy, he recognizes that public awareness is ahead of the science. The result is that the demand for services has outpaced the availability of experienced physicians willing to treat the disorder. He receives calls and emails from physicians and parents all over the country who are seeking his expert guidance, and he feels a responsibility to guide the field with scientific rigor and knowledge. Keeping up with the patients, the inquiries from physicians, the research, and developments in the field can be challenging. He said he understands that busy pediatricians who are seeing patients every fifteen or twenty minutes do not have the luxury of reading some of the more arcane literature. As an example, he referenced a recent article that he had read in the Journal of Leucocyte Biology about, "white blood cells (B cells), receptors and TLR-activated expression of CLIP. So who is going to read that?" He asked. "I barely have time to read the literature," he added.

Dr. Geller would like to develop a systematic approach for physicians of what is needed to diagnose PANDAS, with criteria that will enable the diagnosis to be differentiated between Definite, Probable, Possible, and Not Likely. It has been difficult both to find psychiatrists interested in treating children with OCD and to find funding for the needed studies. He would like to be able to create a national registry where the types of pertinent data for diagnoses are collated and outlined along with how to set thresholds of treatment. He worked with Tanya Murphy, MD in 2012 to develop a study designed to measure not only the response of children with PANS to antibiotic treatment, but also to detect pathogenic agents and markers of immune function.

Dr. Geller feels the onus is on physicians to do a careful clinical inquiry, which means digging into the child's pediatric medical records. If parents do not arrive with the full set of pediatric records and a comprehensive history of the child's medical care, Dr. Geller will make the appropriate requests of pediatricians and then dig in with his highlighter. It often takes at least a week for pediatric records to be delivered to him. He thinks it would be "wonderful" for parents to follow my recommendation to come to appointments fully prepared with all the needed information in hand. What he needs are the key pieces of information that will enable him to determine whether there is a temporal (time-linked) association between the infection and the onset of abnormal behaviors. When I asked him if there was a particular red flag that alerts him to PANDAS, he said, "early age onset and dramatic onset, and possibly new onset urinary symptoms." He also said he sees more anxiety and OCD than tics.

Ideally, Dr. Geller wants to know, "When were the throat cultures done? What did they show? What antibiotics were prescribed and taken over what period of time? What was the response?" He said it's not always possible to provide all of this information because 40% of strep infections are clinically silent, but making a timeline of the records is important. He said the same is true of mycoplasma, which can cause children to be sick with walking pneumonia, but there can also be much milder cases that might be passed off as a cold or cough. Important pieces of information may become apparent by thoroughly reviewing the pediatric records and listening to the caregivers. "Most clinical stories have fragments of information that are suspicious or indicative, but don't allow a definitive diagnosis," said Dr. Geller, "such as a history of low grade fever or minor illness associated with onset." A second area of interest for Dr. Geller is the history of the family as a whole. In particular, a family history of autoimmune disease or anxiety is often present. "I think it's our responsibility to document as clearly as we can all of these factors and to weigh them and to give a judgment," he said.

The easy cases are the ones where blood work shows a massively elevated titer. In the cases where the titer is elevated but not extreme, it's difficult to draw a firm conclusion because pediatricians are not routinely drawing anti-strep antibody titers so there is no baseline to reference. Then there are the cases that appear to be PANDAS, yet the titer is only marginally elevated or it may be within the normal range. Dr. Geller is looking for the clinical signs of PANDAS in all cases, but the clinical observations become particularly important when the serum antibody or immunoglobulin are not elevated. Can the rapid onset of behaviors be linked to an infection? Is there a history of previous lesser behaviors? Was there an earlier period when the child was inexplicably anxious, had difficulty with schoolwork, did not want to separate? Was there a temporal association between the child's behaviors and recurrent nose infections, strep in a sibling, an ill parent, or perhaps a friend who was sick a great deal? When did the child start repeatedly blinking his eyes or twitching his neck? What is the history of autoimmune disease in the family? The answers to those questions may lead him to believe that PANDAS is probable or possible. He would prefer to have an elevated titer or a positive culture to corroborate those cases; but in those more complex, multilayered situations when he feels it is a probable or possible case of PANDAS, "I'm likely to err on the side of treating because I think the treatment risk is low. I don't have solid scientific evidence in those cases," said Dr. Geller, "what I sometimes have is a convincing history of response to antibiotic treatment."

When Dr. Geller treats a PANDAS case, he uses a "robust" dose of antibiotics, using the recommended treatment dose or higher and not prophylaxis doses. His first choice for treatment is Augmentin when the suspected pathogen is strep. If the child does not respond, then he will try a different antibiotic such as azithromycin. Typically, he sees a response within two to three weeks. He will also prescribe traditional psychotropic medication to address the psychiatric symptoms as needed, but generally not concurrently to allow antibiotics a chance to work and before committing a child to an extended (6-12 month) course of SSRI's. Each case is different, but his first choice will be one of the SSRI or Prozac family of medicines that have been shown to help OCD symptoms in children. Typical doses and guidelines may be found in the American Academy of Child and Adolescent Psychiatry,

"Practice Parameters for the Assessment and Treatment of Children and Adolescents with OCD" (J. Am Acad Child Psych 2012).

I told Dr. Geller that I've received many inquiries about vaccinations. He said that clinical experience shows that in PANDAS children, vaccinations could aggravate the symptoms via activation of the immune system. Nonetheless, he does NOT advocate missing the routine scheduled vaccinations recommended by the American Academy of Pediatrics and as guided by pediatricians. Elective vaccinations, for example with the flu vaccine, require a risk benefit analysis that must be made for each child, except for children with asthma or pulmonary conditions where it is usually recommended.

Dr. Geller is certified in psychiatry and child/adolescent psychiatry by the American Board of Psychiatry and Neurology. He is also certified in pediatrics by the American Board of Pediatrics. Dr. Geller completed a fellowship in developmental pediatrics at the Johns Hopkins University Kennedy Institute for Handicapped Children. Dr. Geller is an Associate Professor of Psychiatry at Harvard Medical School.

ERIC HOLLANDER, M.D.

Eric Hollander, M.D. is Clinical Professor of Psychiatry and Behavioral Science at Albert Einstein College of Medicine. Einstein is affiliated with Mondefiore Medical Center where Dr. Hollander runs the obsessive-compulsive and autism spectrum program. Dr. Hollander is also in private practice at the Spectrum Neuroscience & Treatment Institute, which focuses on PANDAS, obsessive-compulsive spectrum disorders, and autism spectrum disorders. Dr. Hollander is one of the few physicians who treats not only children, but also adult patients with PANDAS.

In 1986, Dr. Hollander started working with patients who had obsessive-compulsive spectrum disorders. He also started to see people with inflammatory and developmental disorders. He believes there is an important immune inflammatory process that goes on in many neuropsychiatric conditions and that the fields of psychiatry and rheumatology are getting closer together. As part of taking the patient's history, he carefully considers whether there is family history of problems with autoimmune and other immune inflammatory type problems. While he routinely assesses anti-strep antibodies for all patients with OCD, red flags for him are recurrent strep infections, ear infections, issues with tonsils and adenoids, and immune or inflammatory problems either with the patient or the patient's family. In addition to running blood work for strep, he routinely screens for all the co-infections such as mycoplasma pneumonia, Lyme, and borrelia. He also looks for blood measures of inflammation.

Dr. Hollander speaks of different, "symptom domains." Repetitive behaviors are a compulsive symptom domain, which he also refers to as a core domain. The other type of symptom domains that often co-occur with the core domain are attentional issues (ADD-like domain), motor tic related behaviors, mood instability, tantruming, disruptive behaviors, and developmental issues or problems with peer interaction or social cognition. He carefully considers whether the history indicates an onset, worsening, or improvement of behaviors that can be tracked to an illness or inflammatory process. For example, he might wonder whether the timing of a child's onset of separation anxiety or fear of strangers can be linked to when someone in the family was sick. Treatment will be differentiated depending upon the symptom domains with which the PANDAS patient presents.

Dr. Hollander treats a wide range of patients. He finds that parents are now very attuned to PANDAS. As a result, they bring their children to him at an early stage for care. Young adults who recognize they may not have been appropriately diagnosed in the past are seeing him, too. PANDAS is also being considered by Dr. Hollander for adults with developmental disorders who have marked changes in their behaviors at different times. For example, he will consider PANDAS if a patient with high functioning autism periodically regresses or has more behavioral problems.

If a patient has elevated strep titers and some evidence that it could be associated with behavioral issues, Dr. Hollander treats with high dose (1000mg) Augmentin XR two times a day for a minimum of three months. He then assesses whether there is a reduction in titers or an improvement in behaviors. Sometimes strep can stay in the tissues of the tonsils and it's tough to eradicate. For that reason, he works closely with an ENT. If the patient has sleep issues or adenoid problems, the ENT may recommend removal of the organ.

Dr. Hollander has seen encouraging results with young adult and adult patients. He sees a number who have literally been so incapacitated that they have been unable to leave the house for years, and often their blood still tests very high for strep antibodies. It is more difficult—but not impossible—to treat them because the disorder has become ingrained, often changing brain circuitry, so they require a more integrated approach. The immune inflammatory process must be managed, coupled with aggressive cognitive behavioral therapy, psychotropic medication, and possibly deep TMS (transcranial magnetic stimulation). TMS targets particular brain areas with electromagnetic pulses that can activate or deactivate brain circuits. TMS treatment is daily for six weeks and gradually decreases to a maintenance program. While these patients are more difficult to treat than children and require a great deal of hard work from both doctors and patients, Dr. Hollander has seen many of them recover and do well.

Dr. Hollander is unique among PANDAS physicians because he is also exploring the "hygiene hypothesis." As more fully explored by Paul Patterson in his book *Infectious Behavior* (see Chapter 15, *Research & Resistance*), the hypothesis is that our increasingly clean environment may be affecting development of the immune system. In its simplest terms, perhaps there is a correlation between the rise of behavioral disorders in developed nations and lack of exposure to conditions which were historically prevalent. Such correlation has been demonstrated with other inflammatory conditions such as Crohn's disease. The "hygiene hypotheses," as it potentially relates to PANDAS, stems from threads of observation in a couple of related areas.

One is known as "fever response" in autism. When a patient with autism is physically ill, the symptoms of autism can dramatically improve. Eye contact improves, and they are generally more engaged. It appears that this happens because the immune system is functioning differently due to the introduction of an infection. Dr. Hollander finds that the most improved symptoms seem to be disruptive and compulsive behaviors.

Another principle involves clinical observations about rural populations in Iowa during the 1940's. When farmers moved off their pig farms to the city they developed multiple autoimmune problems: rheumatoid arthritis, asthma, thyroid illness, inflammatory bowel disorders, and MS. When they moved back to the farms, they improved. Similarly, it is widely noted that children who grow up on farms have less issues with allergy and asthma than their urban counterparts. At the University of Iowa in the early 2000's, Joel Weinstock, MD, whose background is in immunology and parasitology, theorized that perhaps the problem wasn't something the farmer acquired when he moved, but rather something he'd lost: parasitic worms (also called helminths). The concept of Helminthic therapy evolved. In this therapy, a harmless parasite is introduced in the hopes that it may reduce the inflammatory response. Dr. Weinstock conducted research using Helminthic therapy for treatment of various inflammatory bowel conditions such as Crohn's disease, colitis, and inflammatory bowel disorder.

In the meantime, a determined father named Stewart Johnson was researching how he might help his violent and aggressive 13 year old autistic son. He came across Dr. Weinstock's work and wondered if it might help his son. The doctor he turned to for help was Eric Hollander. Dr. Hollander knew that some helminths have evolved over time to live in balance with the human system and can serve to dampen down the inflammatory response. He also believed there was a link between autism and the immune system. Dr. Hollander was open to Mr. Johnson's thoughts and, after careful research and consideration, he agreed to a trial of Helminthic therapy for Lawrence. The results were stunning: Lawrence's violent and aggressive behaviors disappeared.

Dr. Hollander used Trichuris suis ova (TSO) to treat Lawrence. TSO is the egg of a pig whipworm that will stay in the stomach for a couple of weeks and is then excreted out, so TSO must be reintroduced every two weeks. TSO do not multiply in the gut or go through the intestines, so they do not cause the problems that are associated with human parasites. Dr. Hollander is now running a TSO trial study for patients who have an autism spectrum disorder with compulsive features. Thinking ahead, he believes that perhaps, someday, Helminthic therapy may be applied to modify the immune systems of PANDAS patients.

Dr. Hollander is certified by the American Board of Psychiatry and Neurology. He is also a fellow of the American College of Neuropsychopharmacology. The Spectrum Neuroscience & Treatment Institute is located on Fifth Avenue in New York City.

RICHARD LIVINGSTON, M.D.

Richard Livingston, M.D. practices child and adolescent psychiatry in Fort Smith, Arkansas (on the Oklahoma border). Over the years, Dr. Livingston has treated hundreds of children with tics, OCD, and hair pulling. He has been treating PANDAS patients since 2000.

Dr. Livingston is the Medical Director of a free standing psychiatric hospital that is part of Vista Health Services, a mental health services organization. The organization offers acute inpatient (hospitalization), residential, and outpatient services throughout western Arkansas. Almost all the hospital's beds are reserved for children, and it is open for admissions 24/7. Ft. Smith is Arkansas's second largest city and is medically sophisticated, but Vista Health services a large, rural area and Dr. Livingston is the only child psychiatrist in the region. Because of the nature of Dr. Livingston's acute care practice, he rarely sees children in the early stages of any mental health disorder, including PANDAS. Children with crisis level behaviors are transported to the hospital for admission either by ambulance or by their parents. Outpatients are generally referred by primary care physicians or schools. He will occasionally be referred a child at an early stage due to an abrupt onset of behaviors, but that is not the general pattern. Generally, the children he sees are incredibly ill with overwhelming symptoms, and he is left to sort out whether at one time in the past there may have been an abrupt onset of behaviors. A further factor affecting his practice is that, in rural areas, families often do not call a doctor unless they perceive an illness to be extremely urgent such as a very high fever or a child who has stopped eating entirely.

Dr. Livingston was immediately fascinated by PANDAS when he first came across it in medical literature. He was initially conservative about treatment, prescribing antibiotics only when a clearly abrupt behavioral onset could be documented, but now he checks ASO titers in every new patient who has any kind of repetitive behavior or possible compulsion. He often sees sky-high ASO titers with no known history of strep. Unless the child has an allergy, his "go-to" treatment is, "one of the cillins: amoxicillin or Augmentin." For a child who is penicillin allergic, he tries azithromycin first as it is generally more tolerable than erythromycin. He treats with the recommended therapeutic dose and estimates that antibiotics work at least half the time. He understands the risks of overprescribing antibiotics in the general population, but he feels the benefits outweigh the risks in the children he treats. They do not have trivial symptoms. They are afflicted with massive tics, major compulsions, and may have, for example, become suicidal or pulled out all their eyelashes, eyebrows, and hair (trichotillomania). It is not unusual for Dr. Livingston to see an ASO titer of 1400 to 1800 (keep in mind that below 200 is considered normal). He steers away from PANDAS when the child's behavior is merely disruptive without compulsions or tics, and if it serves a manipulative purpose such as trying to delay a stay in the juvenile detention center. Dr. Livingston also does not suspect PANDAS when the cutting is situational. For example, if a child cuts (slices his own skin) only when in a detention center it is probably not PANDAS. Dr. Livingston will generally prescribe psychotropic medication to manage the psychiatric symptoms. But in those rare instances when he is lucky enough to see a rapid onset case with psychiatric symptoms that are not crippling, he will prescribe only antibiotics.

One of the most interesting correlations discovered by Dr. Livingston is the prevalence of high ASO titers in teen-agers who engage in cutting and other non-suicidal self-injurious behaviors. In 2010, Dr. Livingston began noticing that some teen-age cutters with OCD behaviors had elevated titers. His clinical observations led him to track ASO titers on all cutters, even those who had no other compulsive behaviors. He found that most of them had high titers. For example, during October 2011, seven out of eight teen-age patients who were admitted for cutting had elevated titers. Tracking 100 teen-age cutters, Dr. Livingston reported in the spring of 2012 that two-thirds of those patients had elevated titers. Recovery from cutting includes not only addressing the infection, but also behavioral intervention as there is often peer reinforcement for cutting. Another potential complication may involve an addiction to the endorphins (the body's natural opiate) produced to block the pain of the cut. Each small slice causes the body to release endorphins to block the pain and, if the behavior has been persistent for quite some time, an addiction may develop. To stop cutting, some patients need Naltrexone to block the "reward" center of the brain associated with addiction.

He sees a clear improvement in about half the PANDAS children for whom he prescribes antibiotics. When he sees that, he will prescribe six months worth of medication. But since the children who are hospitalized are so deeply in crisis he expects the children to improve under his care. After all, he has intervened on many different levels: psychotropic medications, antibiotics, and behavioral intervention. The key for him is whether the response is sustained. If the family takes a PANDAS child off the antibiotics or does not refill a prescription, there will ordinarily be a dramatic decline. Ideally, he wants to follow the children every two months and run labs at that time, too. However, often the children are followed by a different doctor once they leave the hospital, so unless the child is readmitted then Dr. Livingston may lose track of the patient at discharge. He tries to have at least one follow up conversation with the treating physician, particularly when the titers are extreme. He explains the basics of PANDAS and directs them to websites and other sources of information. Dr. Livingston generally finds the doctors he speaks with to be open to it, "just puzzled." Their openness may be a function of the rural, relatively poor area in which he practices. Doctors there don't have much time for theorizing, and the patients do not have many options. If there is a relatively safe treatment that works, doctors will go with it of necessity.

He further pointed out that, "most doctors understand the basics of autoimmune illness, it's not a foreign concept to them."

"Except when it comes to the brain." I commented. "There seems to be a large segment of the medical community who understands autoimmune disorders, but when we get to the brain it's different; suddenly it doesn't apply. Why do you think that is?" I asked.

He chuckled, "The brain puzzles everybody."

He thinks it's important not to overlook PANDAS when there are other contributing causes. For example, one of his patients was the daughter of a methadone addict. At 18 months, she was already hoarding food, attacking people, seldom slept and, if she did, would sleep only on the floor of her foster mom's bedroom. She never smiled and made slow progress in therapy. Shortly after her sister came down with strep, the little girl was compulsively sucking her jeans and became a patient of Dr. Livingston. He found that her ASO titer was elevated by fifty points. After four weeks on amoxicillin, she transformed to a happy kindergartener. "When I told her an 'elephant joke' today," Dr. Livingston said, "she laughed like a kid."

Dr. Livingston is encouraged about greater recognition of the disorder because at a recent conference of the American Academy of Child and Adolescent Psychiatry several prominent researchers made it a point to distinguish, "non-PANDAS OCD," in their presentations.

Dr. Livingston is certified in psychiatry and child/adolescent psychiatry by the American Board of Psychiatry and Neurology, and he has been a board examiner in both areas. He has served as the Director of Child Psychiatry at the University of Arkansas for Medical Sciences and at the New Jersey Medical School. He is currently Adjunct Professor of Psychiatry at the University of Arkansas for Medical Sciences.

TANYA K. MURPHY, M.D.

Tanya Murphy, MD is a professor in pediatrics and psychiatry at the University of South Florida's Morsani College of Medicine. It was in my desperate search for answers to Sammy's illness, that I was introduced to Dr. Murphy via email. I had reached out to doctors at major hospitals in Boston and New York only to be told that I was on the wrong path. But when I posed my PANDAS question and theory to her late one night, she emailed back, "I could not agree with you more." Buoyed, I pressed forward.

Dr. Murphy's interest in PANDAS started in 1994 at the University of Florida shortly after she finished her training in child psychiatry. "I was in the right place at the right time," she said, "because there were a number of experts in rheumatic fever and strep there." The UF team was intrigued by the recently published study from Susan Swedo, MD of the NIMH reporting a correlation between strep and OCD. They decided to further explore Dr. Swedo's work. Funded by a grant from the OC Foundation in 1995, Dr. Murphy began her PANDAS research. It quickly became her passion. In addition to treating children with the disorder, Dr. Murphy is one of the foremost PANDAS researchers in the country. She has authored 140 publications.

Dr. Murphy has treated hundreds of PANDAS patients. Most of the children she treats end up functioning much better. Some fully recover with a complete remission. She believes the extent of recovery may be tied to the patient's level of an antibody to carbohydrate A. This carbohydrate is the "A" in group A strep and may drive the body's autoimmune reaction. Dr. Murphy theorizes that the antibody to carbohydrate A may be acting as a stimulator or neurotransmitter, causing the production of too much dopamine in the brain. There is no commercially available test for this antibody, but she has found elevated levels present in the children in her research studies.

Dr. Murphy estimates that her office is seeing three to six new patients a week. When a child has acute, overnight symptoms, she tries her best to see them quickly because she knows that early treatment produces the best results. About two-thirds of her patients are from Florida, but parents have brought their children from as far as California, Kansas, Missouri, and Oregon. "I've been working in psychiatry for 20 years, and I've never seen psychotropic medications turn a child around as quickly as I've seen antibiotics turn a PANDAS child around," said Dr. Murphy. She has seen the symptoms of children with the severe, overnight, terrifying onset of OCD behaviors come down to nothing within a few days of starting antibiotics. For that reason, she believes antibiotic treatment should be explored first.

In reliance on her clinical gut, her first choice of antibiotic is Augmentin when the presentation is tics. For acute, severe OCD presentations, she will prescribe azithromycin and has found mycoplasma present in many of those cases. Dr. Murphy prescribes within the upper limits of the clinical range and stays with it for at least three weeks to see if she gets a response. Most children will respond within those three weeks and, if they don't, she might prescribe it for a longer time or may switch the patient to a different antibiotic.

The children need to take their medication every day as prescribed. She has seen flare-ups after missing just two or three doses. She believes the antibiotic must be having a neurological effect through a mechanism of action that has not yet been identified. Parents are sometimes concerned that their children seem, "addicted to Augmentin," because the tics return immediately when the Augmentin is stopped. She prefers to continue the Augmentin for these children, but if parents really want to try stopping, she suggests summer as the best time. There are generally less infections going around and less close contacts. Dr. Murphy also advises to carefully consider your child's activities. "You can't imagine how many kids I've seen with flare ups after crawling around in ball pits at amusement parks," she said.

"There are just so many things that go into this," Dr. Murphy said, "but the idea that people are taking hold of this as a possibility for psychiatric illness, that's real exciting. Even in the early 1990's, a syphilis screen was a routine step in psychiatry for patients with psychiatric symptoms. I don't know how much syphilis is around today, but the point is that it was still in our repertoire to look for physical causes. No psychiatry does that anymore." She pointed out that many psychiatric drugs originated from treating infections. When patients in sanatoriums were treated for infections such as TB, it was noted that their moods improved. They were calmer and less agitated. Those observations opened the door to the exploration of psychotropic drugs.

She feels the complexity of the disorder may make it difficult to sort out and treat for a physician who does not see this often. How long has the patient had the illness? What was the real trigger: strep, mycoplasma, EBV, another infection or the flu? For a physician who does not really know what OCD looks like, or what the tics might be, her advice is listen to what the parents are saying. "When parents say their child is so dramatically different, that this is not like their child, those would be clues to do an infection work up." Dr. Murphy said, "We know there are subclinical infections. We know they drove rheumatic fever in the 1980's. We looked for strep as a trigger for patients presenting with acute carditis, so why not look for it in a patient presenting with acute psychiatric or neurological symptoms?"

Dr. Murphy's overall clinical observation is that strep tends to trigger the tics that have more of a compulsive flavor such as tapping and touching. Simple tics such as nose scrunching, eye blinking, coughing, and snorting seem to be driven more by regular anxiety, an allergy, or a virus. However, she has seen some simple tics that develop overnight such as head whipping be associated with strep in the throat, and subside when the infection is treated.

Dr. Murphy strongly supports the role of Cognitive Behavioral Therapy (CBT) in helping with recovery. While she believes that OCD can be biologically triggered, "it can become so paired with anxiety that the avoidance and escape mechanisms can become habituated." For any child who is at least three years old and has not totally remitted, she recommends CBT to help break the habits. Tics tend to fade with antibiotics, but Habit Reversal Therapy (HBT) is an option for persistent tics in children who are at least eight or nine years old. Younger children have a tougher time with HRT skills.

She urges cautions about the use of IV Ig because the children relapse with only one treatment. She's observed that some children do better after three treatments, but they have, "by no means remitted." She feels IV Ig is not appropriate unless the children can be defined as immune deficient or there is otherwise biological evidence that warrants the treatment. It's invasive and incredibly expensive. Moreover, multiple IV Ig treatments, particularly when given every four weeks, can result in hyperviscosity, a thickening of the blood. When faced with a child who has 'through the roof' behaviors then she feels all options must be explored. Absent those dire circumstances, Dr. Murphy feels there must be more research as to how much, how long, or when in the course of treatment IV Ig is appropriate. Even when children do improve with IV Ig, Dr. Murphy feels it is unclear if improvement is due to the Iv Ig, the steroid burst given before treatment, or the antibiotics that are now routinely prescribed following IV Ig.

Dr. Murphy is the director of the Rothman Center for Pediatric Neuropsychiatry located at the Children's Health Center within All Children's Hospital in St. Petersburg, Florida. She is certified in child and adolescent psychiatry as well as general psychiatry by the American Board of Psychiatry and Neurology.

CATHERINE D. NICOLAIDES, M.D.

Catherine Nicolaides, M.D. is a developmental pediatrician in southern New Jersey. She is the doctor who diagnosed Sammy with PANDAS and then orchestrated his treatment. Dr. Nicolaides is unusual in that, unlike most developmental pediatricians who are in academia, she had her own practice for many years. She has recently moved her practice to Children's Specialized Hospital in Egg Harbor, NJ. As a developmental pediatrician, she treats the full range of developmental disorders: ADHD, Tourette's, autism, anxiety, pervasive development disorder and so forth. When I took Sammy to see her, she had treated about a dozen PANDAS patients. Since that time, her PANDAS practice has exploded to the point that she now sees about two new PANDAS patients a week.

Formerly, her PANDAS patients were mostly children with years of history making treatment very difficult. The current group of patients tends to have had a more recent onset which, she said, "really makes it a lot easier to treat." More times than not, the children's parents have figured out their children probably have PANDAS. "They are coming to see me because they've read *Saving Sammy*, been in touch with you, or been on the website and found the information," said Dr. Nicolaides. "Nine times out of ten, it's because of the tireless work you've done, and we all thank you."

The earliest PANDAS case she recalls treating involved a boy who displayed ADHD symptoms and exhibited extreme school phobia. Dr. Henrietta Leonard and Dr. Susan Swedo had spoken at a recent conference she had attended. Their presentation caused her to correctly consider PANDAS in this boy, who then fully recovered on antibiotics.

A more recent case is that of a child with conversion disorder who presented with pseudo-seizures and school anxiety. He failed to respond to traditional psychotropic medication. She began to wonder if the conversion disorder might be linked to a strep infection, although he had been treated for a couple of infections with various antibiotics during this period. Nonetheless, she sent him for a throat culture. It came back positive. Dr. Nicolaides prescribed a high daily dose of 2000mg of Augmentin XR (extended release) twice a day. Within days, the pseudo seizures subsided, and he went back to school. Dr. Nicolaides made no changes to any other medications, so she knew the Augmentin had produced the response. Once recovered, when she tried to discontinue the Augmentin, his symptoms returned. She immediately resumed the Augmentin and, once again, he responded.

PANDAS may present primarily as OCD and/or tics, but it will often be accompanied by other symptoms such as separation anxiety or urinary problems. She finds that the children who have true Tourette's generally do not have other symptoms such as anxiety or enuresis. She looks at all the symptoms to help decipher what's going on, "but most of it is in the presentation. It tends to be an explosive onset that comes out of nowhere, or multiple symptoms all at one time, to the point where it's fairly debilitating." Uncontrollable movements, separation anxiety, enuresis, and getting "stuck" in an OCD way are all red flags for her. When it's unclear, if it's been there a long time, or if the parents are not particularly good historians, she looks for other signs. Constant motion may be one of them. Sometimes children are referred to her for an ADHD evaluation, but when they have nonstop, uncontrollable movements she wonders about PANDAS. She recalls a boy who could not keep his hands still, even when he tried sitting on them. He had some of the other ADHD symptoms in addition to irritability, but no sign of strep. However, when he repeatedly failed to respond to traditional ADHD medications, she decided to try Augmentin. He responded. Another boy sent to her for an ADHD evaluation had a rash on his chin. His mother said it came from chewing on his clothing and drooling. Dr. Nicolaides thought that the rash looked suspicious. Reviewing his medical history, she noted he'd had impetigo. Impetigo is caused by strep. She sent him for a strep test. When it came back positive, his pediatrician was stunned.

In prescribing Augmentin, Dr. Nicolaides agrees there is a dose relation in terms of age, weight, and height. "I just think it's higher," she said mentioning a recent bulletin to pediatricians indicating that increases across the board might be warranted. For a four to six year old, she'll probably start with 600mg liquid Augmentin twice a day; childhood age (eight to ten or twelve years old), 875mg twice a day; beyond that she'll prescribe pills of 1000mg, 1500mg or 2000mg twice a day depending on the situation. The extended release Augmentin is preferable, but only comes in 1000mg pills. She will start with the lowest dose. If she does not get a response within a week or two she will try a higher dose before she abandons treatment. This is especially true when she has tried traditional (psychotropic) medication and sees no response. She will also increase the dosage if there is a partial response, but debilitating symptoms remain. When the children do respond to Augmentin, it usually happens within a few days. She told me sadly that she has not observed that same sort of dramatic response to the antibiotics she must prescribe for children who are allergic to penicillin (Zithromax, Clindamycin, or Omnicef). "The secret is in the Clavulanic acid," she said. Clavulanic acid is part of Augmentin.

Dr. Nicolaides believes the children require maintenance antibiotics. The length of time will depend upon whether the child presents with a new onset of symptoms or a chronic case, and the severity of the symptoms. Generally, after two or three months, if the child is doing well, she will try weaning the dosage, but not stopping it. A child on 2000mg might be reduced to 1500mg and then remain there for an extended period of time. If there is an exacerbation of symptoms, then the dosage will go back up. It's the same approach she uses with psychotropic medications. As an example, she gave a hypothetical child being treated with SSRI's. Once the behavioral symptoms are in remission, generally prescribing physicians will not suddenly discontinue the medication. The dosage will be incrementally decreased to see whether there is a relapse of symptoms. Dr. Nicolaides believes that for purposes of this disorder, the antibiotic should be titrated and withdrawn similarly to psychotropic medications. She also mentioned that sometimes a child on a maintenance dose will still get a strep infection or another sickness that results in an exacerbation. She will usually wait to see if the child can ride it out before increasing the dosage, but sometimes an increase is necessary.

Dr. Nicolaides attended Hahnemann Medical College in Philadelphia. Her pediatric residency was completed at New York University Hospital. She then completed her Developmental Pediatric fellowship for the first year at Johns Hopkins Medical Center and the following two years at Children's Hospital of Philadelphia.

ROBERT SEARS, M.D., FAAP

Robert Sears, M.D. (Dr. Bob) is a pediatrician in private practice in Capistrano Beach, California. The Sears Family is known for its many pediatric publications and its "AskDrSears.com" website. Dr. Bob began treating PANDAS in 2010, and has seen less than a dozen PANDAS patients so far with the disorder. Dr. Bob considers PANDAS when a child who was behaviorally or developmentally "normal," presents with a sudden onset of different behaviors. Examples include OCD, tics, tantrums, oppositional behaviors, or a loss of ability to concentrate at school. Typically, he runs ASO and Anti DNase-B titers as well as takes a strep throat culture. If the labs are abnormal, he will treat with antibiotics. The children's responses have varied. Some did well on just a couple rounds of antibiotics. Others have struggled, some having been unable to maintain despite a variety of treatments including antibiotics and steroids. In one case, the child's titer simply won't budge. Stomach related side-effects can complicate treatment when they are severe enough to warrant backing off the antibiotics.

Dr. Bob is frustrated because initially a large segment of the medical community was in denial that PANDAS was a legitimate disorder. Now that more are acknowledging it, he's still not receiving any guidance from medical organizations on how to treat PANDAS patients. He thinks it may be ten or twenty years before the body of mainstream research is extensive enough to satisfy the American Academy of Pediatrics, the American Medical Association, or the American Academy of Child and Adolescent Psychiatry. He believes that only then will treatment guidelines be offered.

Dr. Bob addresses the infection by prescribing the full therapeutic dose of antibiotics for about a month. If there's an improvement, Dr. Bob will continue the prescription for three to six months and sometimes longer. If he doesn't see an improvement, he may change the antibiotic to see if he can find one to which the child responds. He has prescribed Augmentin, Zithromax, and Omnicef. He has also used oral penicillin once a week, with a penicillin shot once a month, as an easier way for the body to tolerate long-term antibiotics. He has not seen more success with one antibiotic over another, and he sometimes sees no response at all. He may also prescribe steroids.

Dr. Bob has what he believes are logical approaches, but cautions that he simply has not treated enough PANDAS patients to be able to evaluate the results. Dr. Bob thinks the children may improve with a gluten and casein free diet. Many children can be sensitive to gluten and casein even with normal testing so, although he will test, he prefers to evaluate based upon whether the change in diet results in a behavioral response. He thinks this is particularly important for children who have either chronic constipation or unhealthy (loose) stools. Because it's possible that strep may be living in the intestinal tract, he suggests depriving the yeast and bacteria of the sugars they need to thrive; in short, starve them. A yeast free diet does not mean that the child just stops eating foods with yeast; the child must also stop eating foods that feed the yeast: juices, sugars, junk food, foods containing artificial colors and additives, and simple unhealthy carbohydrates.

If the child has a yeast overgrowth, he will prescribe Nystatin. Nystatin can safely be taken for many months without any worry about side effects. Probiotics should be taken when on antibiotics because they help the good bacteria to thrive. He cautions, however, to carefully read the ingredients on the label. Some probiotics contain strep species and although it may not be the same strep as that causing PANDAS, it's best to steer clear of any strep at all. If the child has diarrhea, it may indicate that the steps you're taking to protect the intestinal tract are not enough. In that case, stool tests may be warranted to detect yeast overgrowth and bacteria called C. diff (clostridium difficile). C. diff can cause severe diarrhea and other intestinal disease when antibiotics wipe out the good bacteria in the gut. If not identified and treated, C. diff can sometimes lead to colitis.

Another aspect Dr. Bob considers is anti-inflammatory treatments, helping the immune system to calm down so that the extent to which the body is responding to the strep is limited. The most potent way is with steroids, but long-term steroids are not an ideal treatment due to side effects. Short-term steroids from five days up to three or four weeks are safe and well tolerated. At some point though, the child will have to come off the steroids, so the patient will need more natural anti-inflammatory treatments that can be taken long term. One natural anti-inflammatory is a high dose of fish oil. According to Dr. Bob, the child should take 2000 to 3000 milligrams of Omega 3 fats. By looking on the label, you will be able to see the amount of Omega 3 per capsule and be able to figure out how many capsules are needed to reach between 2000 and 3000 milligrams. Another natural anti-inflammatory is the Indian spice Turmeric. The active ingredient in Turmeric is Curcumin. For this, Dr. Bob recommends a supplement called Enhansa that he describes as well respected.

He knows there is a place for psychiatric medication to control the symptoms while the infection is being addressed. As a pediatrician, he has very little training and almost no experience with these medications so he will involve a child psychiatrist. The involvement is not to clear up the diagnosis, but rather to address that needed aspect of patient care. He has seen the appropriate use of psychotropic medications really help some of his patients.

Dr. Bob supports vaccinating healthy children and routinely administers vaccines in his office to children of all ages. In children who are predisposed to an autoimmune reaction, such as PANDAS, he feels parents must carefully weigh the benefit versus the risk. Whenever you have a child with a severe autoimmune neurological disorder, especially if you've gotten them to recover, he feels you must be very careful not to do anything that might trigger an abnormal autoimmune response. For that reason, Dr. Bob will usually recommend ceasing vaccines for any child with a significant psychiatric or neurodevelopmental problem. And because autoimmune reactions from vaccines are generally more common in teenagers than in younger children, the teenage group may warrant even more careful consideration.

Dr. Bob is board certified and a Fellow of the American Academy of Pediatrics. He is a co-author in the Sears Parenting Library, including The Baby Book and The Portable Pediatrician, and is the sole author of The Vaccine Book and The Autism Book. He is an editor for AskDrSears.com.

ROSARIO TRIFILETTI, M.D.

Rosario Trifiletti, M.D. (Dr. T) is a pediatric neurologist who practices in Ramsey, New Jersey. In 2009, he opened a practice devoted exclusively to treating PANDAS patients. He estimates that he has treated more than 1000 such patients since that time. While the vast majority of the children he treats are afflicted with strep, Dr. T subscribes to the broader definition of PANS. This is because he has treated some children whose behaviors have been triggered by other infections, too, such as mycoplasma and Lyme. Dr. T was one of the first physicians to actively begin looking for mycoplasma in PANDAS patients.

The red flag for Dr. T is the acute onset of any type of behavior. When a new patient sees him, he orders blood work and instructs the parents to start administering ibuprofen right away, as if the child had a fever of 104°. During the week while he waits for the results of the blood work, the parents keep track of whether the child responds. Usually within that week, there is some improvement. The blood work he orders includes Group A strep, mycoplasma, Lyme, and IGG testing. He also orders ceruloplasmin, seritin, and vitamin D, which are acute phase proteins that should rise with a fever or inflammation. When the levels are low, he often sees improvement by adding iron and Vitamin D to the diet. For strep, he will prescribe Augmentin up to double the recommended dose. If the patient is allergic to penicillin, he will prescribe a cephalosporin. Mycoplasma he describes as, "much more tenacious," because it lacks a cell wall and must be treated with a macrolide such as erythromycin or clarithromycin. Dr.

T said that just as the flu peaks every year, mycoplasma peaks every four to seven years. Some children may require both antibiotics if they have both infections.

For a "pure strep" patient, which is mostly what he finds in young children, he recommends removing the tonsils. He describes a tonsillectomy as a bloody operation and handling that tissue, potentially laden with strep, can cause the bacteria to disburse throughout the system resulting in a post-op behavioral exacerbation. For that reason, ten days before a tonsillectomy, he will start the patient on clindamycin in an effort to sterilize the tonsil tissue prior to surgical removal.

Dr. T's usual course of treatment will begin with three months of antibiotics to treat the infection. If he gets no response, he may then try a "steroid burst" to reduce inflammation. A "steroid burst" is a high dose of steroids for a few days. If the child still does not respond to either antibiotics or the steroids, then he is inclined to believe that the child is suffering with genetic OCD and he probably cannot help that child.

Dr. T said that ninety percent of the time, PANDAS/PANS can be treated with antibiotics and mild anti-inflammatories without the need for IV Ig or plasmapheresis. He will ordinarily suggest IV Ig only when he has tried antibiotics for about six months and sees some response, but feels it should be better. He said he has learned that if the children take steroids prior to IV Ig it will help avoid the headache, which is often caused by the sudden flood of proteins that the procedure sends to the brain. According to Dr. T, it is only a handful of patients who will need plasmapheresis.

He has observed and agrees with others who have suggested three categories of children with the disorder: (1) Infant/preschooler who present as super hyperactive and are often misdiagnosed with ADHD; (2) Juveniles who have an acute onset and the child changes virtually overnight; and (3) Adolescents who are doing well in school, suffer a severe infection such as appendicitis, experience acute anxiety, possibly develop chronic fatigue, and may never make it to college.

Dr. T theorizes that while healthy immune systems respond to infections with inflammation and fevers, those whose immune systems are compromised may respond behaviorally. In essence, he thinks that almost any infection that can give children fevers may potentially be able to produce symptomatic behaviors. He believes this, "alternative fever response," may be a malfunction in the branch of the patient's immune system that addresses allergies. "Think of the immune system as the entire United States defense system with its many different branches." He said. "If you knock out one branch, you can survive; but with one branch knocked out - let's say the navy - it's hard to win a war."

What he finds striking in his PANDAS patients is blood work pointing to a low histamine state. This indicates that the allergy reaction is shut off. I asked why histamine is important. "Histamine is one of the neurotransmitters in the brain," he answered. "With a low level of histamine, too much serotonin, dopamine, and norepinephrine (brain chemicals) are produced, and not reabsorbed properly, so you end up with a chemical storm in the brain. That's what PANDAS is, a chemical storm."

A low histamine state is detected when blood results show a triad of low IGe and IGg4 (both antibodies involved in the allergy system), and basophils. Basophils are the main source of histamine in the body and form a portion of the body's white blood cells. Interestingly enough, in the New England Journal of Medicine on May 20, 2010, researchers reported they had found the gene for Tourette's. The gene contains the enzyme that causes the production of histamine. Tourette's patients lack the gene that enables production of histamine throughout the system. Many of the behaviors of PANDAS patients - such as tics - are described as being similar to Tourette's behaviors.

If Dr. T's theory is correct, it may explain why a PANDAS patient will often suffer with even more behaviors when prescribed a Selective Serotonin Reuptake Inhibitor (SSRI). An SSRI slows down the chemical reabsorption (reuptake) process, leaving chemicals in the brain for longer periods of time. Due to the low histamine state, the chemical balance is already off. The SSRI forces those chemicals to remain in the brain even longer.

I know without a doubt that an SSRI can be a big mistake for a PANDAS patient because I watched what happened to Sammy. He never improved at all when he was prescribed an SSRI, he only grew worse. At one point, he even had me ask the prescribing psychiatrist if the SSRI could be causing his behaviors.

Dr. T said that histamine is very closely related to the sleep system, which is why PANDAS children may have sleep disturbances.

The low histamine state may also explain why PANDAS patients do not respond well to antihistamines. An antihistamine (for example Benadryl) turns off the production of histamine, tampering down the allergic reaction. But what a PANDAS child needs is more - not less - histamines in the system. Reducing them even further only exacerbates the storm taking place in the brain. Histamine is also closely tied to the eating center which he feels may explain why anorexia plagues some PANDAS children.

"What will raise the histamine level?" I asked Dr. T. "Parasitic activity will raise it," he answered. This may explain why Dr. Hollander's autistic patient responded to TSO therapy. "It's hard to think about giving children worms, but that will definitely raise histamines," Dr. T added.

With early intervention, appropriate treatment, diligent monitoring, and careful management of exacerbations, Dr. T feels that the children and their immune systems will recover. But they need antibiotics along the way because, he said, "the best way for an army to recover is to stop the war." Once the child makes it through puberty, "something magical happens," he added optimistically, and the recovered children's immune systems do not appear to suffer long-term damage.

As far as vaccines for PANDAS children, he feels parents must carefully weigh the risks and benefits. Some of his PANDAS patients who were vaccinated for swine flu had severe exacerbations a couple of weeks after receiving the vaccine. Regarding boosters, he suggests having the PANDAS child's titers measured to determine whether a booster is really needed. Most children will have received all of their vaccines for pneumonia before they are two years old, but if your child's vaccine was delayed and he now has PANDAS, have a careful conversation with your doctor. Pneumonia and strep are closely related. Dr. T feels that the HPV vaccine may not be the best choice for a PANDAS child, so he suggests thoroughly discussing it.

In late 2011, I referred a patient to Dr. T who had just been hospitalized for the fourth time at a regional psychiatric hospital that is unfortunately full of nonbelievers. The child's mom emailed me the night before the admission to ask if I had any thoughts. Her son had repeatedly tested negative for strep. Following my advice, she had his blood drawn on the way to the hospital and tested this time for mycoplasma and Lyme. Three days later she emailed, full of hope. The Lyme wasn't back yet, but his titer for mycoplasma was off the charts.

"I often wonder," Dr. T subsequently emailed, "how many children in psychiatric hospitals have this condition."

Dr. Trifiletti is certified in pediatric neurology by the American Board of Psychiatry and Neurology.

CONTACT INFORMATION

FOR THE PHYSICIANS WHO SHARED
THEIR VIEWPOINTS ON TREATMENT

David Band, MD
Crossroads Psychological
Associates
10774 Hickory Ridge Road
Columbia, MD 21044-3646
410-992-7288

20905 Professional Plz # 220
Ashburn, VA 20147-3409
(703) 858-9841

Ali Carine, DO
Integrative Pediatrics
3300 Riverside Drive, Suite 200
Upper Arlington, Ohio 43221
614-459-4200

Daniel Geller, MD
Director, Pediatric OCD Program
Massachusetts General Hospital
Child and Adolescent Psychiatry
Yawkey 6A
55 Fruit Street
Boston, Massachusetts 02114
(617) 724-6300 x133-1056

Eric Hollander, MD
PANDAS Center
901 Fifth Avenue
New York, NY 10024
212-873-4051

Richard Livingston, MD
10310 Mayo Drive
Barling, AR 72923
479-494-5700

600 S. McKinley Street
Suite 300
Little Rock, AR 72205

Tanya Murphy, MD
University of South Florida
Rothman Center for Pediatric
Neuropsychology
800 6th Street South
4th Floor, Box 7523
St. Petersburg, FL 33701
727-767-8230

Catherine Nicolaides, MD
Children's Specialized Hospital
6016 Black Horse Pike
Egg Harbor Township, NJ
08234-9701
609-645-7779

Robert W. Sears, MD, FAAP
26933 Camino de Estrella
Suite A
Capistrano Beach, CA 92624
949-493-5437

Rosario Trifiletti, MD, PhD
246 N. Franklin Tpke.
Suite 5
Ramsey, NJ 07446
201-236-3876

WEBSITE REFERENCES

The following key websites relate to material presented in this book:

Beth Alison Maloney's websites:

www.savingsammy.net

www. pandasfoundation.org

National Institute of Mental Health

PANDAS/PANS
http://intramural.nimh.nih.gov/pdn/web.htm

Director's Blog
www.nimh.nih.gov/about/director/2012/from-paresis-to-pandas-and-pans.shtml

International OCD Foundation

www.ocfoundation.org

Rogers Memorial Hospital

www.rogershospital.org

Cunningham Panel

www.moleculera.com

Columbia Mouse Study

www.mailman.columbia.edu/news/antibodies-strep-throat-bacteria-linked-obsessive-compulsive-disorder-mice

Infectious Behavior by Paul Patterson, PhD

https://infectiousbehavior.wordpress.com

Sugar as the Worm on the Hook for Bacteria

http://blogs.discovermagazine.com/80beats/2011/05/12/sugar-helps-antibiotics-kill-dug-in-bacteria/

Walk-in Labs for Blood Work

www.anylabtestnow.com

For continuous updates, visit Beth Alison Maloney's Facebook fan page. You do not need to join Facebook to view the page. You can click through by visiting the Links tab on www.savingsammy.net.

INDEX

Acknowledgments

I wrote this book for you at my desk, at my kitchen table, on airplanes, in courthouse lobbies, during breaks at the UC Irvine PANDAS conference, on trains going back and forth to courtroom battles in Boston, and in college libraries while my son James toured the campuses. Parts were written at my friends homes: Sharon Bialy's condo in Santa Monica, Justine Tanguay's camp in northern Maine, and Marty McGannon's lake house in New Hampshire. I wrote during rainstorms, blizzards, on sun splashed days, and moonlit nights. I kept writing whether the material was tough or the words flowed easily onto the page. When I wasn't writing at my computer, I was writing in my head while I was kayaking, cycling, skiing, or golfing (not particularly well). I talked about the writing to my sons, my friends, and my cat. Sometimes, I wrote in my sleep. Years ago, one of the monologue writers for *The Tonight Show* told me that a writer never stops writing. I thought he was exaggerating.

Kathy Abou-Rjaily, who coordinates the PANDAS support groups that meet across the country, is a large part of why this book came to fruition. She devoted a chunk of one summer to helping me rework its structure and became my tireless editor. Without her, it simply would not have happened quite so well. I am forever grateful for her help.

Tristram Coburn, my agent, was always there for me. "Drink coffee," was his cogent writing advice at one point. It always worked.

I thank everyone who read the manuscript at different points along the way: those mentioned above and especially Nancy Kling and Maureen King who came back in for the final pass. Dr. Tanya Murphy was kind enough to review the opening chapters to gauge whether I was on track; reassurance—from such a brilliant researcher and treating physician—gave me confidence. When I decided it was imperative that this be ready for the first Northeast PANDAS/PANS Conference, it was my brother Cris Maloney who guided me with publishing tips.

I wish I could have included more doctors, more researchers, and even more information, but a book has its limits—so does a writer. I am grateful to each of the doctors, researchers, and others who are mentioned throughout the book, and those not mentioned who are working so hard on behalf of your children. It was an honor to interview many, talk with them from time to time, and include their thoughts: David Band, MD, Michael Baumann, MD, Ali Carine, DO, Madeleine Cunningham, PhD, Stephanie Eken, MD, Daniel A. Geller, MD, Eric Hollander, MD, Peter Lake, MD, Richard Livingston, MD, Tanya K. Murphy, MD, Catherine D. Nicolaides, MD, Paul H. Patterson, PhD, Bradley C. Reimann, PhD, Robert Sears, MD, and Rosario Trifiletti, MD. Kevin Price, MD helped simplify the more complex parts of the medicine. Susan Martin offered her expertise in education. Meg Wolff helped with her nutritional insights.

Writing books is somewhat like launching children. You may wish you'd been able to do more, but at some point you have to trust you've done your best and send them off into the world.

Made in the USA
Lexington, KY
30 March 2018